HOLY & WHOLISTIC HEALTH!

HEALTH PEARLS
FOR THE WHOLE PERSON

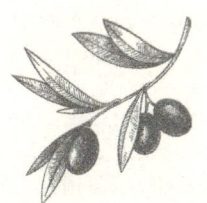

DR. JONATHAN L. CLARK, M.D.

SQUARE TREE PUBLISHING
www.SquareTreePublishing.com
Copyright © 2022 by Jonathan Clark
All rights reserved, including the right of reproduction in whole or in part in any form.
Unless otherwise noted, Scripture quotations marked NKJV are taken from the New King James Version®. Copyright © 1982 by Thomas Nelson. Used by permission. All rights reserved.
Scripture quotations marked NASB are taken from the New American Standard Bible®. Copyright © 1960, 1962, 1963, 1968, 1971, 1972, 1973, 1975, 1977, 1995 by The Lockman Foundation. Used by permission. (www.Lockman.org)
Scripture quotations marked NIV are taken from the Holy Bible, New International Version®, NIV®. Copyright © 1973, 1978, 1984, 2011 by Biblica, Inc.™ Used by permission of Zondervan. All rights reserved worldwide. www.zondervan.com. The "NIV" and "New International Version" are trademarks registered in the United States Patent and Trademark Office by Biblica, Inc.™
Scripture quotations marked ESV are taken from the ESV® Bible (The Holy Bible, English Standard Version®), copyright © 2001 by Crossway, a publishing ministry of Good News Publishers. Used by permission. All rights reserved. The ESV text may not be quoted in any publication made available to the public by a Creative Commons license. The ESV may not be translated into any other language.
Scripture quotations marked NLT are taken from the Holy Bible, New Living Translation, copyright © 1996, 2004, 2015 by Tyndale House Foundation. Used by permission of Tyndale House Publishers, Carol Stream, Illinois 60188. All rights reserved.
Scripture quotations marked KJV are taken from the King James Version, public domain.
Scripture quotations marked AMP are taken from the Amplified® Bible (AMP). Copyright © 2015 by The Lockman Foundation. Used by permission. (www.Lockman.org)
Scripture quotations marked NCV are taken from the New Century Version®. Copyright © 2005 by Thomas Nelson. Used by permission. All rights reserved.
All references to Hebrew and Greek translations of Biblical verbiage are from Blue Letter Bible, https://www.blueletterbible.org/.
For more information about bulk purchases, please contact Square Tree Publishing at info@squaretreepublishing.com.
Cover design by Sharon Marta
ISBN 978-1-957293-08-0

Table of Contents

Preface

Introduction

"In the Beginning" — For Good Health

PART 1 — Background Principles

Deconstructed into Reality — "For Good Health" 23
Journey into Theology — "For Good Health" 27

PART 2 — Practical Observations on Holy Wholistic Health

BREATH
Lungs — "Breath of Life, Breath of God" 43
The Voice — "Exhaling Sounds" 53
Nostrils — "The Fragrance of God" 57
Taste — "The Flavors of Life" 63

BLOOD
Blood of Life — "The Breath and the Bread" 69
Water — "Earth's Elixir and Cleanser" 75
Time-Out — "Holy Wholistic?" 83
Heart — "The Emotions of Life" 87
Blood Pressure — "The Flow of Life" 99
Fun Break — Nerding out on God 111

BREAD
Stomach and Intestines — "The Bread of Life" 117
Liver and Kidneys — "The Inner Man?" 127

BRAINS
Brains — "The Thoughts of Life" 133
Sleep — "Life's Regular Time-Out" 139
Memory — "The Replay of Life" 145

BONES
Bones — "The Framework of Life" 153
Posture — "Upright Living" 155
Muscles — "The Energy of Life" 161
Theology Break 171

BALANCE
Balance — "The Balance of Life" 179
Aging, Reserve, Margin — "The Inevitabilities of Life" 185
Longevity — "The Span of Life" 189
Hormonal Balance — "The Rhythms of Life" 193
Temperature Balance — "The Warmth of Life" 195

BEYOND
Tears — "When Life Leaks" 209
Inflammation — "The Swelling of Life" 215
Relationships — "The Connections of Life" 221
Detoxes — "Life's Cleansers" 231
The Tortoises and the Hares — "Physiological Speeds" 235
Esteem — "The Confidence of Life" 237
Stress — "The Pressures of Life" 241

Final Thoughts 245

Dedication

To the Spirit of God who gives breath to lungs, strength to bones, clarity to thoughts, beauty to sight, pleasantness to fragrances, sensitivity to hearts, understanding to minds, inspiration to ideas, meaning to relationships, and purpose to life.

Acknowledgements

My wife Christa and I are in this together; what I have experienced, we have experienced; what I have written, we have written.

I would also like to thank our kids, grandkids, and family, who always love, accept, and support me; our Abundant Life Church family, who surround and partner with me; the many patients, staff, teachers, mentors, and friends, who continually teach me; and Jesus, who continually changes me.

Endorsements

"I have known Jon Clark for over 30 years, and he is a humble man who 'walks the walk he talks.' As an associate pastor of a local church, as well as a practicing family medicine physician, he has synthesized the most important aspects of 'holy' wholistic health. Being spiritually and medically sound, he weaves the essence of health and biblical concepts throughout this book and makes it both entertaining and easily readable. **Holy and Wholistic Health!** helps the reader discern the important and relevant aspects of health and spirituality together. The concepts put forth make it an excellent read for anyone wanting to truly become physically, spiritually, emotionally, and relationally healthy!"

—Jamie Ulbrich, M.D.
Family Medicine, Past President and Board Chair
Missouri Academy of Family Physicians
Marshall, Missouri

"Dr. Jonathan Clark is a highly creative and experienced father, medical doctor and ordained minister who has captured 'pure gold' wisdom from the world of personal health and healing. **Holy and Wholistic Health!** is a joy-filled masterpiece that springs from thousands of years of the Christian faith and decades of outstanding medical practice. This beautiful conversation with Dr. Jonathan will inspire and challenge you to live the healthiest life in your body, soul and spirit."

—Dave Harvey
Director of Bethel Leaders Network
Bethel Church, Redding, CA

"I have known Dr. Clark for over 34 years. Fortunately, we started our journey together after fully surrendering our lives to the Lord. Dr. Clark doesn't just 'talk the talk' of his faith in Jesus—he walks the walk! After many years of walking together, I had the privilege of ordaining him as a pastor, then later as an evangelist, in our local church.

Dr. Clark not only practices good medicine (he is my go-to medical doctor of choice), but he walks in the Biblical gifts of miracles and healing. I am grateful for the number of times I came to him needing medical treatment, received prayer as part of the visit, and after prayer, discovered I no longer needed the treatment. That's what I call a good doctor!

I anticipate that Dr. Clark's book, **Holy and Wholistic Health!**, will be an encouragement to many, and who knows, maybe God will use it to release miracle health and healing into your life? I pray and expect that He will."

—Benjamin Davis
Lead Pastor, Abundant Life Church
Springfield, Missouri

"I am so honored to present to you a book that will open the door to priceless realization about health and healing for you! Jonathan has bravely shared the inner workings of his mind, soul, and spirit as he leads us through a journey carved out by his medical training, his compassionate physician experience of the spectrum of human emotional expression, and his personal spiritual growth through it all, led by the Holy Spirit. This book is a first of its kind. He provides a series of guideposts, liberally highlighted with scriptural context, to mark the significant points along the way of understanding *truly* holistic health. His incredibly intimate, conversational style will draw you in and make you feel fortunate to be privy to such a private disclosure of treasures that only such an experienced, wise physician and devoted lover of the goodness and power of his divine Father could offer to you. I can only assure you that as you read, you will realize how astoundingly you have been favored to have been given this chance to glimpse many hidden nuggets of wisdom, freedom, and inspiration. Here, we see a true healer who knows and cares for the confluence and complexity of triune humans, created and loved by a triune God."

— Jennifer A. Kang, M.D.
Director, Restore Healthcare Project, Bethel Healthcare Network

"I'm a science educator and person of faith, and **Holy and Wholistic Health!** offers a fresh perspective for communicating the truths of health science and the truths given to us by the God of science. Dr. Clark is both humorous and masterful as he fuses medical science, spiritual insight, lifelong experience, and biblical truth to give readers a pathway on which to travel the journey of "Good Health and God Health." I believe this book will resonate with all those who seek a deeper connection with the practicality of living a healthy lifestyle while enjoying the spiritual victories along the way."

— Linda Underwood
Science Teacher and Dept. Chair
New Covenant Academy, Springfield, Missouri

Preface

As both a family practice medical doctor and an ordained minister, I have witnessed great advances in medical science and increased numbers of miracle healings over the past 30 years. I have seen firsthand incredible medical achievements and supernatural miracles—natural and supernatural solutions. I am so blessed to have multiple vantage points. I love to care for people with all the tools in my tool belt. I am a diligent student of the Bible, science, and medicine—a constant seeker of the Lord and a curious observer of human nature. This is the reason I wrote this book—to share some pearls and tidbits of things I have learned in this process of living and learning, and to encourage people to open up to the realities of holy, wholistic health.

God is not limited to a "one-size-fits-all" healing. He uses medical science, miracles, prayer, emotional healing, natural remedies, and renewed thinking to impart health and wholeness. He is bigger than we think, and He is in the smallest of details.

This book is intended to be a fun read that might also give insights to promote healthy living. I don't claim to be a skilled writer, so please forgive any participles that might be dangling!

One of the greatest things we humans desire and strive for is to be healthy. As is commonly said, if we have good health, we are truly blessed!

I personally think about good health for many reasons. I want to be healthy and live a long, healthy life (especially now that I'm past 50); I want to see my family and friends live happy, healthy lives; and I'm a doctor, and pursuing good health for others is my daily work.

The definition of being healthy—having good health—has many facets and will certainly be defined in many ways by many people. I often hear the term "holistic" as pertaining to health, and I like the term and the concept. It implies good health for the "whole" of man—all of mankind's different parts and organ systems, inner and outer, visible and invisible. Whatever good health may be, I think it must include the wholeness of man.

Holistic is the term commonly used to describe health for the whole person, but "wholistic" is also an accurate term. I like the term wholistic and will use it throughout this book to describe good health for the whole person.

> Bible Pearl:
>
> The word *whole* occurs 240 times in the King James Bible.

As I continually think through and ponder good health, my definition and perspective is from my personal vantage, which is shaped by who I am. As a physician, my definition of good health will contain a scientific and medical aspect. As an ordained minister and a man of Christian faith, my definition of good health will have spiritual and biblical components—thus I will use the term holistic as a play on the word *holy* or *divine* or *God-related*. I have been a doctor, a spiritual person, and a human for a long time, so my unique angle on living healthy will have my experiential flavors added in.

Everyone may not agree with my definition of healthy, and I am okay with that. My purpose in writing this book is to record many observations, tidbits, conclusions, anecdotes, and thoughts on being healthy that have helped me and many others over the years. Some of the observations in this book may be, perhaps, just for my own amusement.

> Note:
>
> I have a dry sense of humor. You might catch glimpses of this as you read through these pages.

There are many good scholarly and scientific books on being healthy written by experts whose credentials are far more accomplished than mine. I apologize to any who may feel that reading through this doesn't add to their practical knowledge base. After reading through this book, at least such a person might know that they have read through health (and theological) observations from another point of view.

In coming up with a definition of what it means to be healthy, I have tried to be thorough and complete, while at the same time being as simple and understandable as possible. Here goes...

From my perspective, living in good health is:

(1) living in a continuous state of energy and vitality.
(2) having the absence of disease and dysfunction.
(3) producing the maximum of well-being now.
(4) experiencing that maximum of well-being for many years to come.

This definition includes maximizing physical strength and functionality and at the same time promoting inner happiness, enjoyment, and peace. It is a state of well-being of the outer (physical) and inner (invisible) person since being human involves both. It is the wholeness of health. It involves vigor. It involves vitality. It involves flourishing. It involves longevity.

A main reason that I wanted to take the time to write these thoughts and observations of good health was to include aspects of my spiritual journey—the Bible, my Christianity, my thoughts on how the holisticness of my Jesus journey has intersected with my enjoyment of the scientific-health world. This intersection of my faith and my field of study continues to produce a perspective on what is whole and holy health. In the following pages, I have separated my thoughts into perspectives on organs, organ systems, and various other health topics. Some of these observations may have practical benefits, and some may just be for my knowledge and/or enjoyment. Whether useful or not, at least I have had fun discovering them as I have pondered health-related research combined with prayer and looking to God and His Word and His spiritual realities.

A primary biblical scripture that addresses the concept of living in good health is one of my favorite verses, 3 John 2: **"Beloved, I pray that you may prosper in all things and be in health, just as your soul prospers"** (NKJV). Other versions say *"prosper and be in good health"* (NASB), *"enjoy good health"* (NIV), and *"that all may go well with you"* (ESV). The writer of this verse, John (of the big three, Peter, James, and John), understood that to live in a state of good physical health was to include the well-being of the whole of man (*as your soul prospers*) and also the well-being of the things and people that are around a person (*in all things*). Wholeness at its finest.

A main concept I would like to pull out of this verse, which will be pivotal to the overall concept of living in good health explained in this book, is the word **soul**—*"even as your soul prospers."* The word *soul* here is the Greek word *psyche* (sometimes seen as *psuche*). This correlates to a Hebrew word for soul found in Genesis, which will be explained next.

Language Tidbit:

When 3 John 2 says, *"be in health,"* John is using the Greek word *hygiano* (Greek was the language of the biblical New Testament authors). Contrasting with the Greek word for healing, *therapeuo*, which focuses more on the act or process of being healed from a disease or affliction (such as in Acts 28:8-9), *hygiano*, where we get the word *hygiene*, focuses more on the state of being well, having soundness, being whole. In the Hebrew (the biblical language of the Old Testament authors), the word *rapha'* correlates with being healed (verb, similar to *therapeuo*), and *marpe'* and *'aruwkah* are both Hebrew words that mean a state of well-being, being whole (Greek *hygiano*).

Note:

The Blue Letter Bible is the source of word translations for Hebrew and Greek.

Introduction

"In the Beginning"—For Good Health

One of my favorite passages in the Christian Bible is the first three chapters, Genesis 1-3, which lay out the Judeo-Christian view of creation and use the powerful first three words of this sacred book, *"In the beginning..."* I believe this book of beginnings contains powerful insights on health and being healthy. I would like to focus on the Hebrew word for soul—*nephesh*—that is used in these early Genesis passages.

As I read the Christian creation story in Genesis, the word *soul* (*nephesh*, sometimes *neshamah*) seems to indicate **the conscious life-force of humans.** Other scientific, religious, or philosophical thoughts may have different words for this—chi, prana, vitality, spirit, energy, pneuma, breath, life-force, and others—but all seem to have at their core a concept of **a conscious essence of life-energy and well-being.**

The concept of soul contains the thought of energy flow (and flow of heat). The human body is made up of atoms and molecules that are constantly experiencing chemical reactions, giving off energy and heat... constantly changing... restructuring...which causes the larger structures (such as organs) to be continually changing and replacing themselves. The physical body, which some consider to be a part of the soul, is a continual flow of physical energy. The essence of the totality of the soul includes the correlating flow of an invisible energy—*psuche* soul energy—that is very real.

> **Tidbit:**
> There are different lines of biblical thought about the interplay of soul and body and how they are related. Some biblical scholars believe that the better interpretation of the original language reveals that even though we tend to separate soul and body for understanding and descriptive purposes, the soul and body are actually one entity. Said another way, no body = no soul; there is no soul without a body; they are intertwined (just like DNA inheritance is intertwined from generation to generation). This is possibly a controversial thought, but the original Hebrew does seem to give support to this.

Back to my definition of good health: (1) living in a continuous state of energy and vitality, (2) having the absence of disease and dysfunction, (3) producing the maximum of well-being now, and (4) experiencing that maximum of well-being for many years to come. This definition focuses all the issues surrounding good health on maximizing all things that enhance energy, strength, and well-being—enhancing what I will call the soul-health (*nephesh*) with its accompanying bodily health. Just as a person's brain is an anatomical physical structure that is visible and must be functioning properly for good health, so too is a person's mind an invisible part of the same person that must also be functioning properly with healthy thoughts for a person to be living in good health. When I use the term *soul* in this book, I am referring to the totality of the human—their visible body accompanied by their invisible correlates.

> **Terms:**
> In the Old Testament (OT) Hebrew Scriptures, soul is usually the term *nephesh*; sometimes *neshamah* is used (perhaps a very important distinction to be discussed shortly). In the New Testament (NT) Greek scriptures, the word soul is often *psyche* or *psuche*.

In Part 1, I attempt to further define and clarify how the human soul/body (*nephesh*) came to exist from a biblical understanding. I believe this discussion will be central to understanding Part 2, which deals with different wholistic (holistic) health tidbits. However, if reading through my more theological-focused explanation of the soul/body is not your cup of tea, feel free to disregard it and go to Part 2. Part 2 is divided into different good health observations based upon bodily organs and organ systems or, in some cases, just based upon a health concept. I do hope you find the following discussion regarding living in good health useful. I suppose we all desire to pursue good health to some degree at different times, realizing that some may be more intentional and serious about health outcomes than others.

*Note: The thoughts and opinions set forth in this book are not to be considered medical advice or diagnosis or treatment. Be sure and consult your qualified healthcare provider for all medical and healthcare advice and diagnosis and treatment.

Wholeness Tidbit:

The New Testament writer Paul touches on the wholeness of man in First Thessalonians 5:23 when he says, *"...and may your whole spirit, soul, and body be preserved..."* In this verse, the Greek word for whole is *holokleros* and is defined as complete and unblemished and sound...whole! Paul brings out the different dimensions of a human and how all dimensions need to be well to experience true wholeness. This line of biblical thought seems to separate spirit, soul, and body as distinct entities, which better aligns with our modern reasoning and rational worldview of splicing and dicing things to help us better analyze and understand them.

PART 1

Background Principles

Deconstructed into Reality

"For Good Health"

I have recently been introduced to a new word—deconstruction. I am familiar with parallel concepts of deconstruction on other levels, such as creative destruction that is always happening around us. For instance, an example of creative destruction in business was when the big box retailer Walmart found a way to do business in a different (creative) way, and this led customers to switch from the smaller mom-and-pop businesses to Walmart. The obvious destruction was the demise of many smaller businesses. Interestingly, in 2020, it was some of the brick-and-mortar businesses that struggled to pivot and became the victims of creative destruction by Amazon and online shopping.

Other historical examples of creative destruction in society: horse-drawn communication being replaced by the telegraph, being replaced by landline telephones, being replaced by cell phones...or Pony Express being replaced by the US Postal Service. Creative deconstruction has formed our history. Airplanes (UPS, FedEx, etc.) have replaced some truck deliveries, which replaced some railroad shipping, which replaced some horse-drawn deliveries. For better or worse, creative destruction is happening around us at all times in different ways.

However, this new concept recently introduced to me is not referring to creative destruction but to the concept of deconstruction—more of a philosophical tool of examining one's beliefs about reality and God, looking for substance and validity and attempting to hold onto only those things that pass the test.

Holy and Wholistic Health!

I reflect on my life and the concept of deconstruction. I was raised in a religious, Christian household with very definite beliefs about reality and God. I was a church-going, good boy with a good quality of life (and was in good physical health). However, over the years as I became a middle teenager, I often felt as though my inner person...my inner man...my soul...was having a hard time breathing. I did not have asthma and did not have any physical respiratory problem, but something inside me was having a hard time catching my inner breath.

So, in the process of time, I turned away from my religious training and my Christian faith. I did not turn to another belief system. Rather, in trying to cope with my inner struggles and inner pain, I deconstructed into a different path, hoping that maybe then I could breathe internally and possibly find a healthier reality.

At first, it seemed to help. I experienced a measure of relief and inner release. But in the process of time, my new reality left me at a place where I had a hard time catching my inner breath and, for the first time, my outer breath. I had spells where I literally couldn't breathe. My new reality wasn't working for me either.

Because of inner pain and symptoms of breathlessness, for survival it was necessary that I deconstruct again and try something different. I would like to say that I went through a slow, rigorous, philosophical process leading me to new solid conclusions about (my) reality. No such luck. My intense inner pain became the cutting edge of my search for a healthy, breathable, peaceful reality.

> **Observation:**
> My inner man was having a hard time breathing in a religious, legalistic system; my outer man was having a hard time breathing apart from God.

Long story short—the breathless spells forced me to talk with someone whom, at the time, I did not want to talk to, but who seemed to be breathing fine. He seemed at peace with the world, enjoying life. I asked for his input and advice and help. His solution—give the Christian faith another

Deconstructed Into Reality

> **Musical Tidbit:**
> One of my favorite songs that epitomizes how genuine this change was in my life is "Abba" by Jonathan David Helser and Melissa Helser. For me, this song describes how Father God and His transforming power were as real as my skin and my bones and the oxygen that I breathe.

try but come at it from a different angle than before. Perhaps the earlier foundation was built on a faulty foundation.

With his help, I gave God and Jesus another try. It worked. I found a new reality and framework for living life and being a healthy, whole person, and this reality allowed me to breathe inside and out. That was 1980, and I was sixteen years old. Since that time, all my decisions about life—regarding family, work, occupation, values, etc.—have developed from this relationship with God and Jesus that made me whole inside and out.

At the time, the pastor at our church often commented that man was a spirit, had a soul, and lived in a body. Interesting. My body and soul in my previous realities were having a hard time being whole and healthy. When I returned to God, it was a spiritual happening. When this third part of humans—the spirit—came alive in me, it made all the difference, and this gave me a useful and healthy reality. I did not return to God because of an intellectual understanding. I just needed fresh air and help. I needed to be able to breathe again. After I started experiencing wholistic health, I decided to journey into an understanding of what had actually happened to me.

In hindsight, reflecting on my return to faith...I returned and found a healthy, viable, thriving faith not through intellectual pursuit but by hanging around others who had a healthy, viable, personal relationship with God. As I observed and experienced others' interactions with God, it rubbed off on me. I found myself experiencing a genuine, truly healthy personal relationship with God for the first time.

Journey into Theology
"For Good Health"

Enter the concept of theology. Theology is the study of God (*theo* = God, and *ology* = the study of). In my former breathless realities, the concept or desire to study God was far from my mind. There was, however, a brief time in my new-found healthy reality in which I considered going to Bible school to be a pastor.

After my transition into peace and healthy living, the person who had previously helped me continued to offer input on my new journey. He became a mentor to me...a discipler (in Christian speak)...a Yoda (in *Star Wars* speak)...a Haymitch Abernathy (in *Hunger Games* speak). This person was also the youth pastor at our church.

After my initial breathing resuscitation, my mentor's recommendation: "Get a Bible and start reading it through. First read through the New Testament and then go back and read the Old Testament. Oh, and make notes while reading." That was over 41 years ago. Since that time, I have read through the entirety of the Bible multiple times. What better place to try to comprehend from a Christian framework the healthy reality that I was now experiencing?

Fast forward more than 41 years—I have been a practicing physician for over 25 years; I have been an ordained minister for over 10 years; and I have been, so far, **living in a state of continuous energy and vitality absent of disease and dysfunction producing maximum well-being** for over 41 years.

I would like to now dive deeper into a few more theological concepts and in so doing attempt to add depth and meaning to what living in holy wholistic health might entail.

In the Beginning...Dust

> *"And the Lord God formed man of the dust of the ground, and breathed into his nostrils the breath of life; and man became a living being"* (Genesis 2:7).

As I have previously mentioned, I love the creation story of Genesis. I love Genesis 2:7 where we get to one of the focal parts—how God brought man to life. But, before we go there, I would like to start at earlier sections and build the story up to this climax of how man came to have a living soul-body that would need good health to maintain and thrive.

Without adding too many references to this discussion and making it cumbersome, I will paraphrase multiple verses in the early Genesis account (feel free to re-read those on your own for review and accuracy). Genesis states that, in the beginning, God created the universe and all that it contains. It further states God formed all earthly things from dust.

When I was a pre-med student, I minored in chemistry and majored in biology. Chemistry was fascinating to me, revealing about the basic elements that make up all matter. I will call all these basic chemical elements, for lack of a better word, biblical dust.

Chemistry has two major divisions—inorganic chemistry and organic chemistry. To help me understand these two divisions, I simplified it

> **Terms:**
> The Hebrew OT term for man is *'adam,* and the term for ground is *'adamah* (notice the resemblance); dust is *'aphar;* life or living is *hay* or *chay.* In Genesis 2:7, the term breathed is *naphach,* nostrils is *'aph,* "the breath" (emphasis mine) is *neshamah* (sometimes spelled *neshama*), soul is *nephesh,* and living being is therefore *chay nephesh.*

down to organic chemistry is carbon-based and the chemical building blocks of all life. Carbon chemistry is the basis for both plant life and animal life. In my mind, then, inorganic dealt with non-life elemental chemistry (biblical dust).

It is interesting to me that the Genesis account says God made life from dust—*'adam* from *'adamah*...man from ground dust. Since carbon is the elemental basis for all physical biological life, He must have used carbon in His crafting of living things; He must have incorporated carbon into His definition of biblical dust.

Regarding God forming the animals, the Bible says God "made" and "created." When He was done with the animals, plants, and fishes, they were alive. They were created living things by God.

In the Beginning...Animals

"Then God said, 'Let the earth bring forth the living creature according to its kind: cattle and creeping thing and beast of the earth, each according to its kind'; and it was so" (Genesis 1:24).

My wife and I are dog people. From the time my oldest daughter was three, we have always had dogs, and it has been interesting studying our dogs in general and the differences in our dogs specifically. It is evident to us dogs not only have a biological physical body, but they also, like humans, have an invisible part, a personality, and the ability to be taught and choose certain behaviors. All of our dogs have been unique.

Interestingly, when the Genesis account talks of the living animals, it often uses the Hebrew word *nephesh*. It seems as though, both experientially and biblically, animals are created with some sort of a soul.

In the Beginning...Humans

*"And the Lord God formed man of the dust of the ground, and breathed into his nostrils the **breath (neshamah) of life**; and man became a living being (nephesh)"* (Genesis 2:7).

Holy and Wholistic Health!

> **Tidbit:**
> Genesis 7:22 also uses the word *neshamah* for breath instead of *nephesh* when referring to the living souls on dry land during the flood of Noah: *"All in whose nostrils was the breath of the spirit of life, all that was on the dry land, died."* The Hebrew translation actually translates "the breath" in this verse as both *neshamah* and *ruach* (a term for spirit that will be further explained)...the breath of the spirit of life...the *neshama ruach chay*...

Animals were created and made and yet have some sort of a soul-body. When God made man from the dust, He went one step further—He breathed (*neshamah*) into his nostrils the breath of life, and man became a living being, a living soul...a *chay nephesh*.

Other Bible versions say a living soul, a *nephesh*. Both animals and humans are called living souls (*nephesh*), yet humans received the breath of life (*neshamah*) as a mouth-to-mouth resuscitation from God Himself.

I apologize if all the Hebrew and Greek words are boring to you. If possible, hold on. I'm going somewhere with all of this.

In God's Image

> *"Then God said, 'Let Us make man ('adam) in Our image, according to Our likeness; let them have dominion...'"* (Genesis 1:26).

When God breathed the breath of His life (*neshamah*)—His Spirit, His wind—into man's nostrils and lungs, man was made in the image of God (see also Genesis 5:1-3; 9:6). There was something in his makeup—his invisible, his soul (*neshamah ruach*)—that was different from the soul (*nephesh*) of animals. Man was made in God's image.

> **Historical Tidbit:**
> In Judaism and in some Christian denominations, only human beings (*'adam*) have immortal souls. Thomas Aquinas attributed "soul" (*anima*) to all organisms but argued that only human souls are immortal (Wikipedia).

The Nephesh Soul 2.0—Upgraded

The breath of God into God's created dust (mankind) gave humans a soul similar to that of animals but upgraded...improved...*neshama ruach*. As the Genesis story continues, it becomes evident that the human soul had been intimately touched by the divine with God's breath, and God is a spirit being. The soul of man had, inbred in it from creation, the ability to not just partake of soul life but also to partake of spirit life. This becomes evident in the creation story; man and woman—Adam and Eve—were able to interact with God in a way that the animals were not. They walked with Him in the garden in the cool of the day...they related to Him...they interacted with Him on an entirely different level.

Adam and Eve—mankind—had spiritual capacity...a capacity to experience spirit life. In my mind's eye looking for a parallel example, I see an image similar to the Coronavirus (I hear groans from the crowd). The structure of the actual Coronavirus is a sphere (soul in my parallel example) that has spikes on the surface (spirit receptors in my example), but unlike the Coronavirus, these

> **Bible Tidbit:**
> *"What is man that You are mindful of him...You have made him a little lower than the angels..."* (Psalms 8:4-5).

receptor spikes are good spikes! As long as humans welcomed the author of spirit life into their existence, their spirit-capacities were activated, and they experienced spirit-soul life in relationship with God. (John 3 speaks of spirit-soul life as being born again.) But, there was trouble in paradise...

The Choice of the Two Soul Trees

When God created His garden in Eden, the one in which mankind was experiencing a spirit-soul life with Him, He put two significant trees in His paradise. One tree—the tree of life—had the capacity to continue to mitigate human's spirit-soul life into an eternal reality.

However, the other tree—we'll call it the bad tree that had a bad infection—was the tree of the knowledge of good and evil. God told Adam

> **Bible Tidbits:**
>
> *"For what man knows the things of a man except the spirit of the man which is in him?"* (1 Corinthians 2:11a). Also, *"For as the body without the spirit is dead..."* (James 2:26).

and Eve if they partook of that tree, they would die. If you know the story, they ate the fruit of the bad tree. They became infected...something in them died...but they didn't physically die at that time. They continued to exist with an invisible soul (*nephesh*). It was now different...changed... dead to the experiential reality of God's Spirit-soul life.

To help understand this concept, and since I am always looking for a relatable example, I see a strong correlation with the struggle between good and evil in the *Star Wars* fantasy series. In the *Star Wars* construct, there are humans who are born Jedi. I would attempt an in-depth explanation of what that means, but I would get it wrong, and my *Star Wars* friends would laugh at me and make fun. Suffice it to say, those who were born Jedi were born with an ability to tap into "the force" and use it either for good (spirit-souls alive to God) or for evil (soul-spirits that are dead to God's life but still have a deformed spirit capacity). Others in the *Star Wars* universe were alive and functioning but did not have Jedi capacity (similar to, in my parallel example, the nephesh souls of animals).

Wow! I read Genesis 3:22 (below), and I realize the overwhelming love and grace of God. What do I mean by that? Man's good spirit receptors were dead, inactivated. But man was still a living soul, just deformed. God, in His great love and mercy toward mankind, did not want them (now in this new deformed soul state that was dead to the ability to interact with God) to reach out and partake of the tree of life and live forever in a deformed, dead-spirit state. Thank you, God, for sending mankind (us) out of the garden!

> **Bible Tidbit:**
>
> *"Then the Lord God said, 'Behold, the man has become like one of Us, to know good and evil. And now, lest he put out his hand and take also of the tree of life, and eat, and live forever—'"* (Genesis 3:22).

Dead to God's Spirit but...

Mankind—represented by Adam and Eve—were now dead to God's Spirit life, but their soul, combined with their flesh and blood, still remained. The Spirit (capitalized S) receptors were dead. However, because mankind was created as a soul-spirit (different from animal souls), there was an "eternal-ness" to their inward makeup.

Eternity in man's hearts. The Bible starts to use the word *heart* for the first time later in Genesis 6 to represent the totality of the inner man. The biblical term heart (*leb* in the OT Hebrew and *cardia* in the NT Greek) begins to represent that man is a soul-spirit...a *neshama ruach*...possessing both a *nephesh* soul and potential spirit (*ruach*) abilities.

> Tidbit:
> *"He has made everything beautiful in its time. Also He has put eternity in their hearts..."*
> (Ecclesiastes 3:11).

Spirit-souls—In the Image of God

Eternity in man's hearts. Humans had an eternal-ness about them from the day God breathed His Spirit-life into their lungs. Mankind, as soul-spirits, after dying to God's Spirit-life, continued to have soul-spirit receptors with the ability to interact with the spirit world. This spirit world was spiritual things not of God.

> Very Important Tidbit:
> Notice that in the term soul-spirit above (apart from God), the soul is first in soul-spirit. When referring to spirit-soul in union with God, spirit is first.
>
> Spirit Tidbit:
> Many believe that the conscience of man is found within man's spirit. Conscience will be discussed in-depth later in relation to good health.

Spirit Things That are Self-focused

Without a long and lengthy discussion about the non-God spirit world, there are a few concepts I would like to bring out. Mankind had fallen for the same seductive trap that fallen spirits had previously fallen for. In God's biblical story, there were and are created individuals who are spirit beings only—angels. When some of the angels (spirit entities without the souls of earthly beings) decided they would prefer to exist apart from God (the Spirit who created them), their eternal spirit nature became deformed, and they decided to eternally exist in a self-focused state apart from God. When Adam and Eve chose to partake of the tree of the knowledge of good and evil, they made the same choice—to live a self-focused soul-spirit life making their own decisions...deciding for themselves what was right and wrong...deciding that God was more of an equal or a lesser... or a non-existent...rather than acknowledging that He was the one who had given them their eternal Spirit-soul in the first place.

In the Genesis story, humans now find themselves outside the garden in their fallen soul-spirit state with eternity in their hearts. The rest of the biblical story plays out with mostly gut-wrenching results until...

Spirit-Soul Life Now Available Again!

Humans did the best they could as soul-spirits, making their own decisions and, at times, using their deformed spirit receptors to interact with non-life-giving spirits. In the fullness of time, God made a way for humans once again to become spirit-soul eternal beings by being in relationship with Jesus, similar to when Adam and Eve originally partook of the same Spirit life in the garden with God.

> **Bible:**
> *"For as in Adam all die, even so in Christ all shall be made alive"* (1 Corinthians 15:22).

Through the sacrificial exchange of Jesus, He who was a Spirit-life generator (Jesus) became a soul man in order that deformed soul-spirit humans could once again be spirit-souls. Those who

> **Bible:**
> *"...The first man Adam became a living being. The last Adam (Jesus) became a life-giving Spirit"* (1 Corinthians 15:45).

receive Him get a reborn newness of life—eternal spirit-souls in relationship once again with the one who breathed Spirit life into mankind from the beginning.

Jesus showed up and made the way for deformed, eternal soul-spirits—devoid of a relationship with their Creator—to once again regain their original design as eternal spirit-souls. Biblically, this is where we are today. All humans are ongoingly deciding whether they will be soul-spirits on their own or spirit-souls with God.

Is This Really a Book About Living in Good Health?

Now that I have briefly given an overview of my theological understanding of the nature of man's soul, I would like to turn back to how to live in good health. I have already given my definition of living in good health as **living in a continuous state of energy and vitality absent of disease and dysfunction, producing maximum well-being now and (hopefully) for many years to come.**

Whatever one's definition of being healthy, it will of necessity touch both the physical, anatomical body and the inner, soul-conscious parts of a person. As I have witnessed repeatedly through the years, a person can physically be in tip-top shape with no diseases and be extremely unhealthy mentally, emotionally, and psychologically. Conversely, a person can be the picture of amazing mental and emotional health and be ravaged by physical disease processes. Good health is both physical and psychological (wholistic), as the original Bible verse that I quoted brings out (holistic): *"Beloved, I pray that you may prosper in all things and be in health, just as your soul prospers"* (3 John 2).

Holy and Wholistic Health!

Wholistic and Holistic Good Health

The remainder of this book focuses on personal tidbits, concepts, and anecdotes that I have observed through the years—observations of humans endeavoring to live in a state of vitality and energy (body and soul), absent of disease and dysfunction (body), with maximum well-being (soul and body) both now (prevention) and for many years to come (longevity).

Most of the time, when we are experiencing good health, we know it. We can feel it. There are times, however, when a person can feel great but have an underlying health problem they are unaware of—a problem that is not yet manifesting in their overall sense of well-being.

> **Bible:**
> *"But if the Spirit of Him who raised Jesus from the dead dwells in you, He who raised Christ from the dead will also give life to your mortal bodies through His Spirit who dwells in you"* (Romans 8:11).

While reading through the remainder of this book, I have inter-mixed what I consider the wholistic (soul-body) concepts with the holistic (spirit-soul-body) concepts. In my mind, because humans were created as spirit-souls from the beginning and this was the original design, wholistic health is truly not "whole-istic" without also including observations of the spirit, observations from the Bible.

The following sections are separated into different bodily systems. However, you will notice as you read through the sections, there is often considerable overlap between the sections and between the different bodily systems. We humans tend to separate things for analysis to aid in our understanding, which is a helpful tool. However, the body itself and the overall whole of man—spirit, soul, and body—are intricately intertwined and function more as "one." I apologize if there is repetitiveness in the following sections.

I hope that you find the following observations insightful and useful; they have been insightful and useful for me. If you do not find them either, at least I hope you find them interesting, possibly even entertaining.

*Reminder: The thoughts and opinions set forth in this book are not to be considered as medical advice or diagnosis or treatment. Be sure and consult your qualified healthcare provider for all medical and healthcare advice and diagnosis and treatment.

PART 2

Practical Observations on Holy Wholistic Health

The following are observations on living in good health—divine health—from the perspective of different bodily organs and systems with (hopefully) some practical applications. Most biblical references will be New King James Version (NKJV) of the Bible, unless otherwise noted. My general framework was based on the question: What things cause energy, vitality, and a sense of overall well-being to increase?

BREATH

Lungs

"Breath of Life, Breath of God"

If you took the time to read Part 1 of the book, which includes the holistic theological framework of humans (a soul-spirit in a body), you may notice some of my observations on the lungs will be repeated. The lungs, in my estimation, cannot be overemphasized, for the lungs were a primary seat of mankind's original creation that set us apart from the rest of all animal life.

I am writing this section while the whole world is in the grips of a coronavirus pandemic. I live in Springfield, Missouri, (United States). Our county had our first confirmed positive case of the SARS-CoV-2 novel coronavirus on March 12, 2020. It has been a year since the first cases were confirmed in China.

> **Bible Verse:**
> *"And the Lord God formed man of the dust of the ground, and breathed into his nostrils the breath of life; and man became a living being"*
> (Genesis 2:7).

At the time of this writing—December 12, 2020—there have been 71,298,626 positive Covid-19 cases reported worldwide, with 1,599,608 reported related deaths. Vaccines are being released, and some are holding their breath (sorry for the pun) to see if vaccines will signal the beginning of the end of this pandemic.

Most of us have never lived through a public health emergency of this magnitude. References and comparisons are regularly drawn to the Spanish Flu pandemic of 1918-1920, in which it is reported that 500 million people were infected, and it is estimated that between 17-50 million people died as a direct consequence of this deadly infection.

With all intention of avoiding the controversial issues surrounding the current coronavirus outbreak, I would like to delve into more of the physical manifestations of someone being infected by SARS-CoV-2 (Covid-19). What we do know so far is its symptoms may vary greatly. Some, especially the young, may have no symptoms or minimal symptoms (like a cold or mild flu). Others, especially those who are older and those with underlying health problems, may develop more serious symptoms.

The list of reported Covid symptoms is long; but for the majority of the critically ill patients—those who may require hospitalization or even intubated ventilation and for those who might eventually pass away—the dangerous symptoms are usually related to the lungs and breathing.

I have a friend who was released from the hospital after receiving ICU ventilation for Covid; another friend who is still on assisted-ventilation after being intubated for a month (hopefully she will make a full recovery); another friend, who was released a month after being on the ventilator, who now says he is still having spells of shortness of breath; and many other friends who have been infected but have fully recovered and have no lingering symptoms of Covid, and their lungs and their breathing have returned to normal.

After Covid passes through an infected individual's upper airway (nostrils or mouth), gets inhaled deep into the lungs, and sets up a Covid respiratory syndrome, some of the pathological manifestations may be similar to other deep non-Covid respiratory infections, such as bronchitis or pneumonia (coughing, wheezing); however, this pandemic virus often follows different physiological pathways that show up in non-typical ways, such as an infected person experiencing difficulty breathing, stating, "I can't catch my breath."

If the shortness of breath continues to deteriorate, the Covid-infected person may have to go to the hospital for oxygen assistance. If the breathing continues to deteriorate on oxygen, the breathless person may have to be

Lungs

intubated and set up on a ventilator...a respirator...a machine that breathes for you when your own respiratory efforts are not working.

Breath of Life

Bible Verse Repeated for Emphasis:
"And the Lord God formed man of the dust of the ground, and breathed into his nostrils the breath of life; and man became a living being" (Genesis 2:7).

Recently as I was reading Genesis 2:7, I realized that mankind's very life essence came when God breathed through his nostrils into his lungs the very breath of life. This was the first mouth-to-mouth (mouth-to-nose) resuscitation...the first assisted-ventilation. As was previously discussed in Part 1, this set humans apart from the other animals, giving them a living soul that had the ability to interact with God's Spirit.

Another Verse:
"The Spirit of God has made me; the breath of the Almighty gives me life" (Job 33:4).

Song Tidbit:
A popular Christian song "Great Are You Lord" by All Sons and Daughters has set to music a lyric about how God breathed His life into us.

I have found it interesting that if Covid infects an individual to the point of potentially dying, it is often because they have lost the breath in their lungs—the seat of their original created life.

Breathing Tidbit:
The lungs are responsible to extract oxygen from the inspired air, a process called ventilation. Once the oxygen enters the bloodstream and into red blood cells, it is transported to all of the body's cells and released into the cells. Once inside a cell, it can be utilized to make energy in the form of ATP. This is called cellular respiration—true respiration—which happens at the cellular level to produce energy and other necessary molecules.

Holy and Wholistic Health!

Check this out: The Bible has different words for breath. In the Old Testament Hebrew language, the word *rua* (*ruach*) is often used to depict breath or wind or spirit. The equivalent New Testament Greek word for breath (spirit, wind) is *pneuma*. What I find incredibly interesting is that the Bible words for breath and wind are also synonymous with spirit. It is God's breath...God's wind...God's Spirit that God deposited in our biological lungs.

I have also found it interesting that one of the main public health mitigation measures to try to contain this virus is to wear masks over the mouth and nose. Again, I will intentionally attempt to avoid the controversies surrounding masks. I will point out that it seems as though this deadly pandemic is attacking at the very Spirit-life (breath) source of humans, and, therefore, some of the public health measures (masking) have had to deal with the gate to our lungs—the nostrils primarily and the mouth secondarily. Both the nostrils and mouth will be addressed separately in further sections.

One of my friends who was recently on a ventilator in the hospital asked me regularly to pray for him. As the doctors and nurses physically gave him life-saving assisted ventilation—THANK YOU, THANK YOU, THANK YOU—my prayers focused on all that could help his spirit-soul bring him back to good health with energy and vitality and an overall sense of well-being (and in this case not dying). My prayers spiritually aligned with what the healthcare workers were already doing. My prayers were, "God, it's Your breath in his lungs, it's Your breath in his lungs..."

Tidbit:

I have a friend who was on assisted ventilation for many days due to a non-Covid-related health problem. Statistically, she had a 90% chance of not living. When the ventilator was stopped and the breathing tube removed, she immediately gasped for air...and lived...and eventually went home. Later, when she was telling me about the experience, she said that she knew that God was the one who breathed His breath of life back into her lungs when the breathing tube was removed.

Lungs

> **Jesus Breath Tidbit:**
> Just as "in the beginning" God breathed His breath of life into mankind and they became spirit-souls (Genesis 2:7), in the New Testament Jesus breathed His new creation Holy Spirit Spirit-life into His disciples, and they became born again in the image of God—fully alive spirit-souls. *"...He breathed on them and said to them, 'Receive the Holy Spirit'"* (John 20:22).

Why not assist and turbo-charge the physical ventilators with the original source of spirit-soul life—the very breath of God—through prayer?

When I asked one of the Covid-veteran ICU nurses about my friend's chances as he went on the vent, she said in her experience only about 25% of Covid-ventilated patients live. When I called back the next day to check on my friend, the good nurse said he was responding atypically—in a good way. Within three days, he was extubated and taken off the ventilator! Approximately two weeks after coming off of the ventilator, he was released to go home, and though he still required supplemental oxygen and was not completely out of the woods, he was much improved. "God, it's Your breath in his lungs...it's Your breath in our lungs..."

Long Covid and the Breath

For those who have been infected with the Covid virus and survived, many have fully recovered with no ongoing symptoms; others continue to experience residual symptoms (at some level). This has been termed long Covid. I am not an expert in acute Covid or long Covid; many others have studied long Covid with good data and understanding.

When I do read about the syndrome called long Covid, it seems as though at least three areas are often involved: the strength (energy and muscles), the brain (brain fog, sleep, anxiety, mental/mood issues), and the breath (shortness of breath and other

> **Tidbits Reiterated:**
> *"The Spirit of God has made me; the breath of the Almighty gives me life"* (Job 33:4). God's breath—God's Spirit—is the very air in our lungs.

lung sequelae). Other symptoms and organ systems may be affected by long Covid, but these three areas stick out to me as being most significant. As most of the health topics discussed in this book will overlap with other chapters, I will address long Covid in more detail in a later section regarding muscles and energy.

Do You Mind If I Smoke?

> **Breathing Nugget:**
>
> "The alveolar membrane is a gas exchange surface, surrounded by a network of capillaries. Across the membrane oxygen is diffused into the capillaries and carbon dioxide released from the capillaries into the alveoli to be breathed out" (Wikipedia).

The lungs are obviously necessary for life. The tissue and cells that make up the lungs are on one hand resilient and on the other hand delicate.

The lungs breathe in air with its normal concentration of atmospheric gasses including oxygen and nitrogen (and others). Mixed in with every breath of air is anything else that is in the air such as pollution or smoke. The air mixture ends up crossing into the body at the end of the pulmonary tree at what is called the alveolar membrane. The alveolar membrane is the lining of the lung cells, the lung cells that some might say looks like a cluster of grapes on a vine.

> **Smoke This?**
>
> It is generally agreed upon in most health circles that cigarette smoking is bad for your health. Not only can smoking lead to emphysema (COPD) and lung cancer, smoking also increases the risk of heart disease, stroke, and other cancers and has been implicated as a factor in many other disease processes.
>
> **But It's a Plant...**
>
> Tobacco is a plant that grows on the leaves of the tobacco plant; therefore, it's healthy, right? No. There may be some as yet undiscovered health benefits of tobacco leaves, but setting them on fire and breathing the smoke into the lungs is not one of them.

> ### All-Natural Goodness:
> I'm all for all natural things in promoting good health. However, all natural and plant-based doesn't automatically make something healthy. Some of the most dangerous and lethal chemicals known to man come from the ground.
>
> ### The Great Debate:
> Many have quit smoking by turning to e-cigarettes and vaping, believing that these are healthier than smoking tobacco. As more time has passed and more research has accumulated, it appears that smoking any other non-tobacco chemical into the lungs is also not healthy and can lead to harmful health problems.

The alveolar lung tissue that comes into contact with air (and other chemicals) is designed, when working properly, to successfully process over 20,000 breaths per day that an average person breathes. Lung tissue is designed for normal air gas concentrations but not designed to handle the "extras" that often seep into our breaths. Carbon monoxide... cigarette smoke...e-cigarette smoke...recreational smoke...many forms of air pollution...toxic odors...It seems as though the lungs are designed to thrive on air and air only. Carbon monoxide poisoning is lethal. Most other forms of ongoing smoke inhalants will eventually lead to lung malfunction, damage, and disease.

Asthma vs COPD

Asthma is defined as a reversible tightening of the airways in response to a trigger, such as pollen, mold, pollution, dust mites, chemicals, tobacco smoke, humidity changes, and many others. The constricted airways can be opened back up by removing the trigger and possibly adding some temporary medication until the airways are fully open. Inhalers and steroids are common treatments when someone is having a breath-stealing flare-up of asthma.

Holy and Wholistic Health!

Any natural-based or soul-based or spirit-based interventions that can help the lungs, the breath, the breathing, are recommended and welcomed to help restore lung and breath function so that people can live in a state of energy and vitality with the absence of disease and dysfunction producing maximum well-being now and hopefully for many years to come!

Miracle Lung Stories:

I have a friend who has the genetic lung problem cystic fibrosis (considered to be incurable) who received a lung transplant along with lots and lots of prayer; she is doing very well. I knew another friend who was a long-term smoker and developed a large lung cancer tumor and was given 4 months to live; she chose to not receive any standard treatment but did receive prayer; she lived at least another 5 years. Every time they re-checked for the tumor, it was still there. When she did eventually pass away, it was reported to me that she died of other causes.

And Another:

While on the topic of miracles, a totally unrelated story. I have an alcoholic friend who was on Hospice and considered terminal with alcohol-related liver damage; he was wasting away and appeared to be on his proverbial last leg. He quit drinking alcohol and in very short order was off Hospice and gaining weight and has lived many years since. I found it pleasantly ironic when he eventually came back in to see me due to the chronic lifestyle problems of weight gain and high blood pressure and high cholesterol.

Just One More:

A friend of mine had an ugly mole on the side of her forehead which did not appear to be dangerous. She wanted it removed for cosmetic purposes (understandably so). We referred her off to a surgeon for removal and prayed for her before she went (at her request). She called me back after some weeks, before seeing the surgeon, and told me that she woke up one morning and the mole was gone!

Lungs

Chronic Obstructive Pulmonary Disease (COPD), otherwise known by the slang emphysema, is a process that has led to non-reversible lung damage. The damage often comes by the ongoing and continued inhalation of chemicals such as cigarette smoke. Some treatments can be helpful and make improvement but, by definition, the damage is not reversible and will not be 100% normal again. I have seen patients with COPD improve after they stopped smoking (everything) and gave it time...

The Voice

"Exhaling Sounds"

Humans have the ability, if they choose, to make their exhaling respirations pass over their vocal cords in such a way as to produce sounds. If they have trained their sounds to be intelligible to others in the form of words, it is possible to communicate with the voice by speaking to others with words in the form of language.

Revisiting Cellular Respiration

Let's focus back on human respiration for a moment. The atmospheric air that we breathe is approximately 21% oxygen. There are other gasses we inhale into our lungs, mostly nitrogen. However, it is the oxygen, the product of green plants given off during photosynthesis, that we need to support our biological life.

Biochemically, we are carbon-based life forms. We already have the carbon, which is supplied to us from our food. When humans breathe by inhaling air, we pull out the oxygen and use it to make energy in the form of a molecule called ATP; ATP is a product of respiration in our cells. The process of forming ATP energy requires taking carbon-based food (primarily in the form of glucose) and combining it with oxygen to produce ATP, heat (body temperature), water, and carbon dioxide.

When we exhale, we breathe out a modified mixture of gasses that now includes a higher level of carbon dioxide. Exhaling is how we remove the not-needed carbon dioxide out of our bodies and send it back to where

Holy and Wholistic Health!

> **Bible Tidbit:**
>
> The Bible verse Nehemiah 8:10b says, "...*The joy of the Lord is your strength.*" This verse has been turned into a popular singing chorus that almost always generates energy in my body as I sing it!

it is needed—back to the plants that will use it during photosynthesis, generating oxygen again in this beautiful and elegant cycle that supports plant and animal and human life.

The molecule carbon dioxide has one carbon atom and two oxygen atoms. When we exhale out carbon dioxide, we are exhaling out carbon...the physical building block of human life.

God's breath (God's Spirit) activated our lungs and continues to sustain our lungs. For this, I will regularly give God my thanks. In one manner of speaking, we breathe in (inhale) the breath of God, the breath of life in the form of oxygen, and we have the option of exhaling our humanity (carbon dioxide) back to Him as vocal praise and vocal thanksgiving. We have the option to breathe in Spirit-life from God and exhale our humanity back to Him in a beautiful flow of spirit-soul-body cycle.

Personal note: Along with all the natural means I use when I am not experiencing wholistic good health, I also have learned to activate my

> **Tidbit:**
>
> When I was infected with Covid-19, I noticed a weakness in my voice—possibly from inflammation in my vocal cord area. I'm not sure if that's common; thankfully it went away quickly.
>
> ....
>
> **Vocal Weakness:**
>
> My mom had Covid at least twice, and I noticed her voice seemed to be weaker than before Covid. Other things that can cause voice hoarseness or vocal cord weakness (to name a few) include laryngitis, vocal cord polyps or nodules (possible from voice overuse or misuse such as yelling or singing improperly), and steroid preparations in the form of nasal sprays and asthma inhalers.

spirit-soul man by turning to God with all of my heart, soul, and strength—including my voice of praise and thanksgiving (holistic). I have found this gives me strength, energy, and vitality in my soul and bodily parts. By returning to God the life He has given me in vocal praise and worship and thanksgiving, my overall sense of well-being, energy, and vitality is enhanced—wholistic and holistic health.

Healthy Words

Do the words we speak have power and influence over our health? Many popular culture books have been written about positive thinking and positive speaking. The Bible seems to bear out the fact that the words that come out of the mouth affect health.

All words are fruit to the hearers. The hearers will taste the words and either accept or reject them. That being so, I want my words to be delicious wine rather than toxic whining; healthy olive oil rather than greasy fat; tasty whole-grain bread rather than unhealthy carbs.

> **Word Health:**
>
> Jesus said out of the abundance of the heart the mouth speaks (Luke 6:45). One of the most impactful verses for my life and health and inner well-being has been Proverbs 18:21: *"Death and life are in the power of the tongue..."*

Everything that comes out of the mouth...words...prayers...songs...confessions and declarations...grumblings and complainings...vile, rotten, foul words...beautiful, encouraging, lovely words...reflect what's currently in the heart and mind and will have an impact on today's health and future health.

> **Heart Murmur Pearl:**
>
> A heart murmur is defined as an abnormal sound that can be heard when listening to the heart with a stethoscope; it is caused by a structural or functional abnormality of the biological heart. The obvious soul parallel—when a person is murmuring with their words, there is an obvious abnormality of their inner heart.

Nostrils

"The Fragrance of God"

Bible Verse Repeated for Emphasis: *"And the Lord God formed man of the dust of the ground, and breathed into his nostrils the breath of life; and man became a living being"* (Genesis 2:7).

The current worldwide Covid-19 pandemic seems to have a predilection for attacking the smell, taste, and lungs. In particular, when trying to symptomatically diagnose the novel SARS-CoV-2 coronavirus, I focus on the symptoms of losing smell and taste because many of the other symptoms are similar to colds and flu, but loss of taste and smell is more specific to this infection.

> **Nostril Verse:**
> *"All in whose nostrils was the breath of the spirit of life..."* (Genesis 7:22). The OT Hebrew word for nostrils is *aph*.

Other than being a double-holed adornment of the exterior human face—with the accompanying outer shell nose that mimics the structure of what lies underneath and is often the brunt of many injuries and jokes—the nostrils are the preferred entry path of human breathing. As air enters the nostrils and filters up through the nasal passages and sinuses, the air is humidified, warmed, and (hopefully) filtered of many dangerous germs and chemicals. Humans do have the ability to breathe through the mouth, but that seems more of a redundant, accessory pathway to be used only when necessary (the mouth has its own specific functions that will be discussed later). If the nostrils and nasal passages and sinuses do their job properly, the natural breath of life (oxygen) is wonderfully presented to

Holy and Wholistic Health!

> ### Smelling Verses:
>
> *"Then Mary took a pound of very costly oil of spikenard, anointed the feet of Jesus, and wiped His feet with her hair. And the house was filled with the fragrance of the oil"* (John 12:3). (See other beautiful Bible verses about fragrant aromas: 2 Corinthians 2:14-16, Ephesians 5:2, and Philippians 4:18).

the lungs in a glorious state of humidified, warmed, partial purity.

In humans, the sense of smell is considered the most primitive, varied, and memory-recalling of the five basic senses. It is intricately involved with the sense of taste, giving all of the tasty overtones and intricacies to the food we eat. The beautiful capacity of smell can immediately take us back to a distant memory that may have emotionally charged responses.

I have a fun little game that I like to play—when I smell honeysuckle, I like to call it Father God's cologne...meaning I know that He is near, and I can smell His presence. I believe He actually is and I actually can!

Humans experience the sense of smell when the aromas in the air—actual chemicals mixed into the air we breathe—pass by the olfactory bulb in the nasal passages. If the chemicals have the ability to produce smell, they are called odorants and will interact with the cells of the olfactory bulb, thus transmitting an interpretation of smell, a sense of fragrance, to the brain for further processing and identification and (sometimes) enjoyment.

Obviously, if an odor is not pleasant, the repulsive smell might be an immediate signal—sometimes even a reflex—that repels us and might warn us of danger. Sometimes a noxious odor can trigger a nausea

> ### Incense Tidbit:
>
> In the OT account of the Exodus, the Lord God was very explicit and specific with Moses about wanting pleasant-smelling incense and anointing oil in His dwelling place, the tabernacle. The expert perfumers were to mix this. Moses was given intricate details about how the incense (perfume) and aromatic anointing oil was to be mixed; the same "holy" mixture was not to be used for everyday perfuming enjoyment (see Exodus 30).

> ### Fragrant Tidbit:
> The sense of smell is considered the most primitive of the five major senses. It develops early in life and has a direct connection to brainstem processing and reflex areas, mostly bypassing the more-advanced intellectual and reasoning areas. Due to the shortcut from nasal passages to the primitive brain, a particular smell can immediately evoke an emotion...perhaps happiness if attached to a pleasant memory...perhaps nausea and disgust and repulsion if attached to an unpleasant memory.
>
> ### Disgusting Tidbit:
> The primitive sense of smell is so powerful that an unpleasant smell can elicit not only horrible memories but nausea and repulsion to the point of disgust. One explanation of disgust is the extreme psychological form of dislike.

reflex. An unpleasant smell may not be dangerous or noxious; we may just not like it.

I have been musing on the fact that the pandemic coronavirus often attacks the sense of smell. One infected person said they smelled a combination of gasoline, mint, blueberry, and pine trees for a couple of hours...and then nothing. No smell. No taste. No enjoyment. Just blandness.

> ### Does That Smell Funny?
> Anosmia is the term for loss of smell; dysosmia is when the sense of smell is altered or abnormal.

Health authorities have recommended humans maintain at least six feet of separation between one another to help prevent transmission of Covid-19 through the air we exhale and inhale. Recently, I was outside and was able to smell cigarette smoke from someone who was at least 40 feet away (to be fair, the wind was blowing in my direction).

> ### Tidbit:
> I recently heard of a preliminary study that seems to indicate that trained detection dogs can smell Covid in the sweat of infected individuals. We'll see if that pans out to be true or valuable.

Holy and Wholistic Health!

> **Lysol Tidbit:**
> During the early months of the Covid-19 pandemic, I was inhaling so much Lysol and air sanitizers—which had a very distinct smell (not pleasant)—that I eventually started experiencing dizzy spells with nausea, feeling off balance and light-headed. It resolved when I started limiting my inhalation of air disinfectants. The malodorous air-sanitizing chemicals were passing through my nostrils into my lungs and into my bloodstream, giving me a symptomatic toxicity. I had to detox off of Lysol for the symptoms to stop occurring.

One of the discoveries about how Covid-19 affects the sense of smell postulated that the virus does not actually damage the olfactory receptor neurons—the smell cells—in the olfactory bulb. It was theorized that the SARS-CoV-2 infects and damages the support cells that are around the cells of smell—cells that are supportive and structural.

I am not a research scientist, but I have often wondered if there is an undiscovered pearl in the sense of smell and the nostrils to fight off or even prevent Covid-19? A nasal vaccine? Something else that is nostril and smell-focused? I don't know. I will continue to ponder this fanciful thought in my free time.

> **Fun Tidbit:**
> Have you ever noticed that when you block one nostril and gently blow... and then block the other nostril and gently blow...that one of the nostrils seems to be a little more open? This is called the nasal cycle, which switches nostrils on average every 2-4 hours, resulting in greater airflow through one nostril at a time. Some have postulated that the nasal cycle also somehow helps with the sense of smell.
>
> **"Funner" Tidbit:**
> The nasal tissue that causes the alternating congestion and decongestion of the nostrils is accomplished by erectile tissue...similar to the erectile tissue found in other parts (ahem!) of the body. Along with the genitals and nostrils, similar erectile tissue is reported to be found in the ear also (insert astonished-face emoji here).

Nostrils

Why Does My Nose Run?

It has been said that the viral cold is the most common infectious illness known to man, thus the term common cold. More than 200 different viruses are known to cause the symptoms of the common cold. An estimated one third of adult colds are caused by a family of viruses called rhinoviruses.

A runny nose is a regular symptom of the common cold and other upper respiratory infections (URIs for short). Seasonal allergies, such as pollen and ragweed, are common causes of rhinitis and sneezing.

Not all runny noses are caused by colds, infections, or allergies. Other forms of nonallergic rhinitis include environmental or occupational irritants, weather changes, certain foods and beverages, certain medications, hormone changes, and sleeping on the back with face and nose up.

> **Nasal Terms:**
>
> The medical term prefix rhino- relates to the nose and was originally derived from a Greek word of similar structure. If the nose is inflamed, it is called rhinitis. The more common use of the term rhinitis is to indicate a runny nose. A stuffy nose can be called coryza. The term catarrh is another way to say excessive secretions in the nose or throat.

> **Fun Rhinitis Tidbit:**
>
> Gustatory rhinitis is the term relating to when a runny nose is caused by eating certain foods, spicy foods being a regular culprit. One source said that gustatory rhinitis is when you experience a thin nasal discharge (the "sniffles") almost immediately after eating a trigger food.
>
> **Another Rhinitis Tidbit:**
>
> According to Wikipedia: "About 50-90% of people get a runny nose when (the weather is) cold. We call this 'cold-induced rhinitis,' or 'skier nose.' Cold, dry air stimulates the nerves inside your nose, which send a message

Holy and Wholistic Health!

> (Cont): through your nerves to your brain. Your brain then responds to this impulse by increasing the blood flow to the nose, and these dilated blood vessels warm the air passing over them. Secondly, the nose is triggered to produce more secretions via the mucous glands in order to provide the moisture to humidify the air coming through."

Smell Your Way to Good Health?

A new word to me regarding smells and health—phytoncides. Not only are essential oils purported to be good for your health, but phytoncides have claims of potentially promoting healthy living.

What are phytoncides? A direct quote from Wikipedia:

> Phytoncides are antimicrobial allelochemic volatile organic compounds derived from plants. The word, which means 'exterminated by the plant'...found that some plants give off very active substances that help to prevent them from rotting or being eaten by some insects and animals...More than 5,000 volatile substances defend plants that protect them from bacteria, fungi, and insects.

It has been hypothesized that being out in nature exposed to trees and plants—what some call "forest bathing"—can increase and bolster certain parts of the immune system. Others tout that being in nature can lower blood pressure and help prevent and maybe even treat many disease processes. There is probably something to that; especially if a person finds being outdoors in nature relaxing, meditative, and enjoyable.

> Note:
> Forest bathing would certainly include breathing phytoncides. Some essential oils might be classified as phytoncides.

Taste

"The Flavors of Life"

As I have previously mentioned, the Covid-19 virus often produces a loss of taste and smell. Bummer. I really like food, and I really like tasting my food. My wife says that I don't actually taste my food since I inhale it so fast. She says I should learn to savor my food. I'm not even sure I know what that means (insert smiley face emoji here).

Many of the younger people I know who have recovered from Covid-19 and experienced minimal symptoms have told me that what they disliked most was not being able to taste their food. When screening patients

> **Awesome Taste Verse:**
> *"Oh taste and see that the LORD is good..."* (Psalm 34:8a).
>
> **Does That Taste Funny?**
> Ageusia is when the sense of taste is gone; dysgeusia is when taste is altered or abnormal.

> **Tidbit:**
> In 2016 my wife and I celebrated our 32nd anniversary on a weekend getaway in Tulsa, Oklahoma. It was February, and I was getting over a common cold. Being a special occasion, we dined at some very nice restaurants. During one of the meals, I realized the food was very bland...so bland that I could not taste anything. The cold virus had made me lose my sense of taste and smell. Fortunately, it returned as soon as my cold went away. In hindsight, I suspect that it was one of the other Coronavirus strains that have existed for quite some time that only cause mild, cold-like symptoms.

Holy and Wholistic Health!

> **A Sweet Verse:**
>
> *"How sweet are Your words (Lord) to my taste, sweeter than honey to my mouth!"* (Psalm 119:103)

and reviewing their symptoms to determine if they have Covid-19, I usually focus on whether they can taste and smell. When they tell me they can still taste and smell normally, sometimes they will jokingly add "unfortunately..." It makes me giggle if it is not a potentially serious situation.

> **A Salty Verse:**
>
> *"Salt is good; but if the salt has lost its flavor, how shall it be seasoned?"* (Luke 14:34)

The sense of taste uses five basic taste buds located on the tongue, which indicate sweet, salty, sour, bitter, and umami. I don't care much for sour or bitter, but I do like sweet in all of its diabetes-causing forms.

Salt is singled out as a flavor-enhancing substance in three of the biblical gospels about Jesus.

It would seem that high blood pressure must not have been a common problem during biblical times with the current recommendation of high blood pressure's low-salt diet. I probably put too much salt on my food, but so far my blood

> **Umami Verse:**
>
> *"He (Jacob) also had made savory food, and brought it to his father..."* (Genesis 27:31).

> **Taste Tidbit:**
>
> I have noticed when I drink coffee, there is a certain temperature range—not super-hot, not lukewarm, somewhere in between—in which my coffee seems to have the best flavor. I have also noticed if food is too hot, I have a hard time tasting the flavor(s). If my food is too cold, the flavors will often be changed and not as enjoyable. I'm sure there are exceptions. It just seems as though many hot foods and hot drinks have a certain temperature range that brings out the best in flavor for my taste buds.

Taste

> **Tidbit:**
>
> Speaking of spices, one spice that I especially like is black pepper. According to Wikipedia, "Ground, dried and cooked peppercorns have been used since antiquity, both for flavor and as a traditional medicine. Black pepper is the world's most traded spice and is one of the most common spices added to cuisines around the world. Its spiciness is due to the chemical compound piperine, which is a different kind of spicy from the capsaicin characteristic of chili peppers. It is ubiquitous in the modern world as a seasoning." My friends make fun of me for over-peppering my savory foods, yet I have yet to find a negative health consequence of the world's most traded spice (except for sneezing when it gets in my nose). Maybe I like pepper so much because one of my childhood pets was a feisty little Pomeranian dog named Pepper; perhaps it was because a high school friend introduced me to over-peppering my biscuits and gravy. I found that culinarily divine!

pressure has remained good. I will continue to monitor my blood pressure closely.

Umami has been described as "savory-ness" and is characteristic of broths and cooked meats. Esau in the Bible used to cook savory wild game, and his brother Jacob got in on his action. Esau's intense desire and love of savory food caused him to sell his birthright to his conniving younger brother Jacob for a bowl of hearty, umami stew.

> **Note:**
>
> Biscuits and gravy is one of my favorite savory breakfast treats that I partake of maybe once or twice a year (well...maybe more). I would love to eat it regularly, but I'm pretty sure my waistline, blood pressure, cholesterol, and heart would not continue to live in good health if I did.

Combined with the five basic taste buds, the ability to smell enhances all the myriads of flavors of foods, adding levels of sensory beauty to our experience of eating...providing enjoyment, pleasure, textures, flavors... the spice(s) of life.

Taste also can have a protective effect by helping us to avoid and spit out foul-tasting food that might harm our bodies. If taste buds help us reject noxious food from passing into our stomachs, our stomachs will not have to violently reject food that has been swallowed. (I don't even like saying the "v" word; it sounds rather vulgar to me.)

> ### Spicy Romantic Tidbit:
> For any who would like extra credit when it comes to the symbolism of taste (and fragrance) and romance in the Bible, Solomon has quite a few racy applications in the Song of Solomon! I won't list those here. You can Google search those or look those up on your Bible app.

BLOOD

Blood of Life

"The Breath and the Bread"

In biological (and spiritual) terms, blood is synonymous with life—no flow of blood, no life.

There are two primary substances that humans require from outside their bodies; there are others but two primary ones I would like to focus on here—oxygen (the breath) and food (collectively I will call food the bread). Both of these external necessities end up in the bloodstream (oxygen in

> ### Interesting Tidbit:
> The OT Hebrew word for blood is *dam*; the OT Hebrew word for man is *adam*. Notice the close interrelated connection between mankind and mankind's blood.
>
> ### Life-blood Verse:
> *"For the life of the flesh is in the blood..."* (Leviticus 17:11a). The blood of all humans and animals sustains their biological life.
>
> ### Life-blood Verse Continued:
> Blood is also the life-force of the living soul and the requirement for a living soul to be made right (whole): *"...I have given it (the blood) to you upon the altar to make atonement for your souls; for it is the blood that makes atonement for the soul"* (Leviticus 17:11b).

> **Tidbit:**
> In Christian terms, bread can be synonymous with Jesus, the Word of God; breath can be synonymous with the Spirit of God (the Holy Spirit). The concept: The Spirit and the Word flow through the blood of life...
>
> ....
>
> **OT Echoes:**
> In the Hebrew scriptures, ingesting blood was strictly forbidden: *"But you shall not eat flesh with its life, that is, its blood"* (Genesis 9:4; see also Deuteronomy 23:25). Blood was considered holy, sacred, pure...reserved for God alone. Fat was also sacred to God; I will discuss it in a later section.

red blood cells and food as fats, proteins, and carbohydrates), where they will be carried to different organs and on into individual cells. The individual cell is where the breath (oxygen) and bread (food) will be utilized.

Don't Go Swimming in the Blood

Individual cells (such as skin cells or liver cells or heart cells) are "where the action is" as far as producing energy, replicating, and the overall business of being alive. A cell is designed to live and exist within an organ or a tissue. Cells thrive and flourish and do their thing within their specific tissue.

The bloodstream—which is the river (so to speak) that meanders through all bodily tissues—is a dangerous place to try to live as a single cell. The environment of the blood is dangerous for a cell unless that cell is a blood cell. And, even then, the blood cells (red blood cells, white blood cells, platelets), which are designed to live in the blood, will not live for long. They are not destined for longevity compared to most other cell types. Between (1) the salty salinity of blood and (2) the liver and spleen constantly filtering and chewing and replacing blood cells, the lifespans of blood cells are relatively short, and their turnover is high. Red blood cells have an average lifespan of about 120 days; platelets last approximately 10 days; white blood cells have a wider range of life, most sources quoting anywhere from 24 hours up to 1-2 months. The three classes of short-lived blood cells are all very interesting in their own special ways.

Healthy Blood Cells or Freakish Martyrs?

Interesting fact: The short-lived and soon-to-be destroyed red blood cells that carry the vital oxygen (breath) are an unusual cell. Unlike normal, non-blood cells, the red blood cell loses its DNA and organelles...it has no DNA once created...kind of like a robot...a mutant (not)...honed-in on one purpose. Some have theorized this design helps maximize the red blood cell's intracellular space for maximum oxygen-carrying capacity.

> **Fun Fact:**
> The salt content (salinity) of blood is 9% compared to seawater's 3.5% salinity.

Another interesting fact: The platelets, the second blood cell destined for a short life (approximately 10 days), do retain some of the regular cellular organelles but have no nucleus...almost like not having a head or a brain...like a zombie, another freakish mutant (not). They are focused on the goal of blood-clotting and minimizing blood loss if a vessel is damaged.

Third interesting fact: The third line of blood cells to go for a relatively short swim (varies 24 hours–2 months) are the white blood cells. Another freakish, zombie-like robot? You be the judge. They have a nucleus that is extraordinarily large and condensed; the nucleus is multilobed (not

> **Tidbit:**
> While most white blood cells are short-lived, the memory B cells and memory T cells (both white blood cells) are on the other end of cellular longevity. Once generated after an infection or vaccination, these white blood cells may last for years. However, they spend their existence stored away in lymphatic tissue such as the spleen or bone marrow (B cells) or in peripheral tissues such as the intestine, lungs, or skin (T cells)—not hanging out and resting in the bloodstream—and can be activated when the immune system is mobilized by an infection.

the norm for cells) with no protein synthesis and few organelles; and the nucleus fills up most of the cellular space (cytoplasm). Another weirdo with a laser-like focus in my observation.

None of the three blood cell lines reflect what is otherwise considered normal cellular structure.

Go With the Flow

The blood must maintain continuous flow with proper concentrations of constituents to sustain life. If it becomes too diluted with water, this equals trouble, possible death to said human. If it becomes too concentrated and/or lacks flow, it will become "sticky" and stagnant and form blood clots and/or lack blood flow, which can lead to death of downstream tissues, and possible death to said human. Blood must flow.

Birth of a Cell

Once the body's specialized organ tissues are established during development, new cells are birthed by replication of the established cells in their tissue. This is mitosis—the scientific term possibly memorized in junior high biology class—which brings about growth and repair. How are the new cells maintained? The flow of blood goes to every cell of the body and feeds, nourishes, cleanses, and detoxes the cell by a sprinkling-bathing effect. Each cell is not submersed in the blood, not taking a swim. The dependent cells require the blood to come and trickle-bathe over each cell, providing each cell with the external needs of the cell.

> ### OT Echoes:
> *"So Moses took the blood and sprinkled it on the people, and said, 'Behold the blood of the covenant, which the LORD has made with you in accordance with all these words'"* (Exodus 24:8 NASB).

To summarize: As a cell, you do not want to go swimming in the hostile bloodstream unless you are a freakish, mutant-like blood cell that has a crystal-clear purpose and no hope of living long.

Blood of Life

> **Pearl:**
> There is a strong symbolic correlation between these observations about blood and tissue cells and the life of a Christian. The Christian believer is considered part of the body of Christ. If each individual Christian correlates to a cell in the body of Christ, the Christian will find their origin and their thriving Christian life—their sweet spot, their place, their reason for being—in a specific tissue (a church community, a group of believers). Their conversion into Christ's body must have the blood (of Jesus) to be birthed... born again...born anew...like the old hymns speak of how Christians are washed by Jesus' blood, making them even as white and pure as snow ("O the Blood of Jesus"). However, if the Christian, the cell in this example, tries to go it alone and jump out into the blood for a swim and try to live solitarily in the life-giving bloodstream of Jesus, they often do not do well...do not thrive...are not robust. They often lack vitality and experience a weak faith... unless they, using the metaphor, are a deformed, mutant-like blood cell with a destiny and calling that is crystal-clear, possibly flaming out in a short life.

Take home point: Healthy blood with healthy breath and bread are essential to produce vim, vigor, vitality, energy, well-being of soul and body for good health and hopefully a robust, long life.

Water

"Earth's Elixir and Cleanser"

In an earlier chapter entitled "Journey into Theology," there is a section called "In the Beginning...Dust" in which I discussed the difference between life-based chemistry and non-life-based chemistry. In a nutshell, life-based chemistry, also known as organic chemistry, is carbon-based, meaning that the carbon atom is a component of all life-based molecules. Organic chemistry was a pre-med requirement, and many of us dreaded this brutal course and simply suffered through it.

On the other hand, inorganic chemistry is the classification of chemistry that is not carbon-based. Inorganic molecules do not contain carbon. Life-containing tissues cannot be built with inorganic molecules alone. Inorganic chemistry is the foundational chemistry course that one might take in high school or college. In pre-med, I found general inorganic chemistry just as difficult as organic chemistry because I had not taken any prior chemistry classes...and chemistry had lots of math and formulas and equations.

> ### Fun Fact:
> My dad was a math teacher and required me to take high-level math classes throughout my school years. I was able to do math, but I did not enjoy it. I was math lazy...until I took pre-med calculus, which is another story for another time. Suffice it to say, calculus was incredibly hard...and fascinating! The concepts were mind-blowing to me. I would often leave class with a headache because my mind was being stretched to new levels.

Holy and Wholistic Health!

Water, Water Everywhere

It is said that the human body is filled mostly with water, some estimates as high as 60% (or even higher). Certain individual tissues contain higher percentages of water—64% (skin), 73% (brain and heart), 79% (muscles and kidneys), 83% (lungs). Even the dry, hard bones are composed of approximately 31% water.

> **OT Echoes:**
> "Then I will sprinkle clean water on you, and you will be clean..." (Ezekiel 36:25).
>
> **Fun Fact:**
> Organic solvents—another category of "dissolvers"—can, as expected, dissolve organic chemicals. A few examples are gasoline, paint-thinner, kerosene, acetone, and ether.

But wait a minute...Water is made up of two hydrogen atoms combined with one oxygen atom (H_2O)...noticeably absent of carbon. Over half of the human body is composed of an inorganic chemical (insert confused-face emoji here). I'll come back to that conundrum.

Another amazing ability of inorganic water is its cleaning and cleansing ability. The chemical properties of two hydrogens combined with one oxygen allow water to function as an amazing solvent, thereby also making water a good cleansing agent.

> **Personal Tidbit:**
> I did research one summer in college as an organic chemistry lab assistant. I spent three hours each day thoroughly cleaning beakers and flasks with soap and water followed by acetone and ether (for chemical purity). Organic solvents are highly volatile, meaning they evaporate easily at room temperature. I spent my afternoons breathing these somewhat floral, somewhat pleasant chemicals. At night, when I would go home with my usual daily solvent-smelling headache, my wife would say she could smell the acetone and ether on my breath for most of the evening as my lungs were slowly exhaling these volatile chemicals out of my system.

Water

The dual action of water-soluble substances dissolving in water and a scrubbing action which dislodges unwanted substances makes water a valuable, easy, and inexpensive natural cleaner. And, if you heat the water, making it a more effective solvent, and add a little soap, it's even better.

Do Blood and Water Mix?

As was commented on in the last section, blood is life. Blood flows through the human body and sprinkle-bathes all the cells for nourishment, cleansing, and detoxing. And yet, blood plasma is 90% water. This amazes me...the greatest part of the soup of life-juice (blood) is an inorganic, non-life molecule. There is a pearl here to be gleaned.

To glean the pearl, let's start with a biochemistry formula (yay! lol), and not just any biochemical formula. Let's look at the chemical equation of how energy is created in the cell, in mitochondria to be specific.

Biology Tidbit:

Mitochondria are intracellular organelles that produce ATP. ATP is the energy currency of all cellular processes. No ATP = no cellular processes such as growth, repair, protein synthesis, and replication = cellular death.

Grammar Note:

Mitochondria is plural; a mitochondrion is a singular mitochondria.

Fun Fact:

The cell's nucleus is the control center of the cell and houses the 46 chromosomes of DNA...kind of like the brain of the cell. DNA on the chromosomes guide the cell's inner workings. Interestingly, mitochondria also contain their own DNA. I'm not sure why, and there are most likely lots of theories. My take—if the nucleus is the cell's brain, all the mitochondria function as the power plant of the cell, requiring its own DNA templates.

Holy and Wholistic Health!

Back to the long-anticipated biochemical formula that everyone is expectantly waiting for (ha!). The formula of how mitochondria produce ATP energy looks like this:

Glucose + Oxygen = ATP + Carbon Dioxide (CO_2) + Water (H_2O)

> **OT Echo:**
> *"So you shall serve the Lord your God, and He will bless your bread and your water; and I will remove sickness from your midst"* (Exodus 23:25).

Glucose, otherwise known as a sugar, contains life-giving carbon and comes primarily from our food; it is combined with the oxygen we breathe (both which are supplied to cells through the watery, saline blood). These chemically interact to produce (1) energy and (2) carbon dioxide (an organic molecule used by plants to produce living substances), and...(3) water...just water...an inorganic compound. Hmm.

For funsies, let me restate the ATP formula in another way:

Bread + Breath (both in the blood) = Energy + Water + Carbon Dioxide

The ATP energy will be used to maximize and maintain good health. The carbon dioxide will pass through the blood back to the lungs to be breathed out as we exhale. The water will be recycled into all of our human biological processes that require water.

> **Interesting Tidbit:**
> When we exhale carbon dioxide, it passes through the air and (hopefully eventually) lodges in the leaves of green plants and is used in the process of photosynthesis. Photosynthesis is essentially the reverse of the ATP-generating cycle in human mitochondria. Photosynthesis takes carbon dioxide, water, and ATP and produces glucose (our food from plants) and oxygen (our breath). This completes one of the most fundamental cycles of life...the carbon cycle...the organic cycle.

Water

Here's the pearl starting to be gleaned: The carbon cycle of glucose and carbon dioxide makes sense (to me). These organic compounds are the building blocks of human life. The ATP makes sense—we must have energy for good health, vitality, and strength. But there are these other two inorganic molecules—oxygen and water—that are intricately and fundamentally and essentially intertwined with all living processes.

In the beginning...dust. God created inorganic heavens and earth before creating all organic life. When He created life, and mankind specifically, He took the dust—the dirt—of the ground (inorganic substances) and breathed His Spirit...His life... His *ruach* (covered in the earlier theology section) into man, and man became a living soul.

> **Pearl:**
> God's design from the beginning was to spiritually and physically intertwine heaven and earth. Without God's Spirit, there is no human soul or human life. Without inorganic dust (water and oxygen), there's no human soul or human life. We "soul-body-Spirit humans" must have water, the inorganic elixir of life, or we don't exist.

Regarding all of our external requirements, humans will physically die quickest without breath (oxygen); after approximately 5-10 minutes, we will have probable brain damage. The next physical necessity is water; it is estimated we can last approximately 3-4 days without water. It is estimated a person can go without food for about 3-4 weeks. (There are reported exceptions to all these general rules.) Oxygen...then water...then food. Spirit...then life-sustaining water... then life-sustaining food.

> **Verse:**
> *"Then God saw everything that He had made, and indeed it was very good..."* (Genesis 1:31).

Water is an amazing solvent and cleanser and a general background infuser of life and health, both inside and outside the cells. For instance, staying well-hydrated during the course of a day is one of the healthiest and simplest things a person can do. When a person drinks mucho agua (I jokingly refer to myself as bilingual; my kids are not amused or impressed), the water rapidly passes through the digestive system and into the bloodstream, expanding blood plasma volume and enhancing blood and water flow throughout the body.

Water flows throughout the body continuously in the bloodstream. Water permeates all of the body's tissues and cells. It's everywhere. As such, water is perfectly positioned to take out the garbage—the leftover cellular debris from regular metabolism—which accumulates as a result of bodily processes.

Said another way—water is one of the primary detox mechanisms of the body. Water (in blood plasma) sprinkles on and percolates to all cells... dissolving and sweeping away unwanted debris into either veins or the

Mega-Health Pearl:

After taking over a medical practice at age 31, I began to work long days in the clinic. I enjoyed my work, *and* it was physically, mentally, and emotionally taxing. I would often notice a late morning lull in energy and a low-grade brain fog. I decided to intentionally start to do something everyone knows is healthy. I decided to stay well-hydrated, intentionally drinking water throughout the day (and avoiding other drinks). An amazing thing happened. My late morning brain fog and overall energy was "healed," and I also noticed that my after-lunch drowsiness was essentially gone! In fact, my overall energy and mental focus increased to levels that I had not previously experienced. Simple and affordable and effective. That's my kind of good health pearl!

Corollary Pearl:

If a person is dehydrated for any reason, low energy, weakness, and fatigue ensue. Whether from illness (such as stomach and intestinal infections) or from exercising on a hot day, there is a direct correlation between my energy levels and the amount of water in my system. A large glass of water at the end of my exercising is immediately restorative. It is designed to be! Heaven and earth coming together.

Water

> **Pearl:**
> The detox power of water is especially pronounced as we sleep (sleep will be discussed in greater detail later). It is theorized that during the deep stage of restorative sleep, the brain tissue contracts...shrinks, if you will...allowing the cerebrospinal fluid (a watery, plasma-like fluid that encompasses the brain and spine) to maximize cleansing flow. This detoxes out unwanted and potentially dangerous, disease-causing brain trash...cellular debris...that might otherwise accumulate in the brain and contribute to or cause dementia processes. Healthy sleep may help prevent dementia!

lymphatic channels, eventually re-circulating toxins and cellular trash back into the full circulation to be excreted out of the body.

Water is Good and Good For You

The flow of water—earth's inorganic elixir that is crucial for human life—in the human body is truly miraculous. It feeds, nourishes, cleanses, dissolves, detoxes, and hydrates. Water is one of the greatest secret pearls producing energy, vitality, strength, good health, and well-being to help remain free of disease for (hopefully) a long life!

Time-Out

"Holy Wholistic?"

Because there is a correlation between water and cleansing and cleaning, I would like to come back to a spiritual correlation of being spiritually clean—the concept of being holy.

Holy Water

The word *holy* and the associated word *holiness* are common words in the Bible, seen repetitively in the Old Testament law of Moses. Holiness is a difficult concept for many to grasp and has been difficult for me as well. What has really helped me to understand this concept more fully is the understanding that the term *holy* in the Bible essentially just deals with being set apart...set apart only for one person or for one purpose and not for anyone or anything else.

> **A Holy Verse:**
>
> "And you shall be holy to Me, for I the Lord am holy, and have separated you...that you should be Mine" (Leviticus 20:26).

Marriage is Holy

The concept of marriage and being wholly (holy) devoted to a spouse is a cultural concept that parallels to being holy or holy unto God alone. When I married my wife, I took a vow of holiness, a vow that I would be wholly devoted to her romantically and intimately (and in every way) and to her only. Now that we are married, I expect her undivided devotion and consecration to me just as she expects the same from me.

Holy and Wholistic Health!

Being only devoted to one person in marriage has helped me wrap my mind around the spiritual concept of holiness unto God. God lives in a beautiful, loving state of clean, pure, holy beauty. It is His nature. It is His essence. For me to be able to interact with Him at any level of relationship, of necessity, I would need some level of holiness (being like Him) to be able to see Him and relate to Him and to be able to interact with Him in any ongoing and meaningful way.

Holy...For Real?

Living in a state of biblical holiness is not as difficult as it sounds; we have added too much religiosity in our understanding of what it would mean to live a holy life. For any Christian who has received the life of Jesus and has a new-life relationship with Him, they have received the sacrificial blood of Jesus applied to their life; Spirit-life with Him is now a reality for them. That person has become a partaker of a new life, a divine nature, a holy nature; it was given to the individual as a gift. By no effort of their own, that person has internally and spiritually been given a holy nature.

> **Divine Verses:**
> *"...(that)...you may be partakers of the divine nature..."* (2 Peter 1:4).
> *"The free gift of God is...life in Christ Jesus..."* (Romans 6:23 NASB).

Because the new Christian has been given a new nature as a free gift, a nature that is internally holy and in union with God's divine holy nature, this new nature (power) enables that person to actually live out externally what everyone would consider a holy life. The new nature is devoted unto God and does not live in biblical or moral unholiness, such as sexual impurity or stealing or killing or vulgar attitudes and words...It is a life of loving and respecting others well in every way.

> **Union Verse:**
> *"...as You, Father, are in Me (Jesus), and I in You; that they may be one in Us..."* (John 17:21).

Time-Out

Said another way, in my own life, any real holiness is generated from the inside out, a free gift from God; the internal holiness motivates and empowers me to live, by gradually being changed over time, in a way that any outside observer might consider to be a holy life. My goal is not to impress others as living a holy life; my goal is to benefit others (and myself) from actually living as a new life person! This is not religion. This is reality and relationship.

Once Upon a Time...

Once upon a time...a man found that he experienced moments of happiness and pleasure...and then many moments of real emptiness and discouragement. This man never knew from day to day what type of day he would experience. This man went all out in pursuit of happiness and pleasure; his highs were high, and his lows were low. His whole pursuit in daily living was to maximize the good moments, however fleeting they may be...and to minimize the empty, shallow moments.

> **Unpleasant Verse:**
> *"Vanity of vanities, all is vanity"* (Ecclesiastes 2:11 NASB).

> **Another Unpleasant Verse:**
> *"So I came to hate life...everything is meaningless—like chasing the wind"* (Ecclesiastes 2:17 NLT).

Over time, this man realized that even during the "good" moments that provided pleasure and some form of purpose, the happiness meter was diminishing. The good times weren't as good as they used to be, and the bad times seemed darker than before. Beauty wasn't perceived as beautiful as it once was.

No big surprise—that man was me in my middle teenage years.

The Beauty and Pleasure of Holiness

Here's the tie-in to holiness—I entered a relationship with the God of the Bible, and my "insides" started to change. Everything started to become different—in a good way. Light became brighter. Happiness became happier. Beauty became more beautiful. Emptiness started to be replaced with purpose and value and substance. My grades in school began to improve, evidence (to me) that I was able to process and think clearer.

What had happened to me? After I entered a relationship with Jesus, I now possessed an internal nature that was a divine (holy) nature, given to me as a free gift. As I nurtured and allowed this wonderful internal new life to develop, I started to live a fuller life…richer…truly more enjoyable and meaningful and more rewarding. And more stable; not as many ups and downs.

> ### Tidbit:
> This true internal fulfillment sort of reminds me of the similarity of when I feel very satisfied at the end of a productive workday.
>
> ### Maybe a Better Tidbit?
> Another example would be the genuine happiness and fulfillment that I have found in my marriage as I have been wholly devoted to my wife in marriage. Holy wholeness has its privileges and benefits! Holy wholeness is good for health!

Heart

"The Emotions of Life"

"Can I do my own heart surgery?"

"Keep your heart with all diligence, for out of it spring the issues of life."
(Proverbs 4:23)

Heart disease remains the leading cause of death in the United States, out-distancing cancer and all other major killers. The term heart disease refers to any disease of the heart. However, when used in modern vernacular, heart disease usually refers to the process of atherosclerosis. Atherosclerosis leads to heart attacks.

> Tidbit:
>
> The fancy medical term for heart attack is myocardial infarction or, if you want to slang it, just say MI. Another fancy medical term for this is coronary artery disease (CAD).

The linguistic definition of atherosclerosis by splitting the word into its two constituent roots is hardening (*sclerosis*) of the arteries (*athero*)...

> Tidbit:
> The medical term that actually means hardening of the arteries is arteriosclerosis. Heart disease that leads to heart attacks is often a conglomeration of hardened arteries over time combined with plaque buildup. Common underlying causes of heart disease—along with older arteries of increasing age—include high blood pressure, high cholesterol, diabetes, and smoking.

athero defined (thank you, Wikipedia) as a gruel-like, soft, pasty, porridge-like material...yuck! Rather than gruel and porridge, the term most often used regarding the heart is plaque. Atherosclerosis is the build-up of plaque (or plaques) in the arteries of the heart muscle arteries, which eventually may lead to a blockage of blood flow through a heart artery. If the blood flow through an artery ceases too long—death to muscle cells downstream—heart attack—MI—myocardial infarction.

A person can have unknown heart disease with plaque build-up in heart arteries but no damage yet, or they may have manifested heart disease with previous heart damage. Standard recommendations for heart disease are to control blood pressure, lower cholesterol and triglyceride levels, maintain normal blood sugar and body weight, and do not smoke (anything). Practical lifestyle habits to accomplish these goals include eating a healthy, plant-based diet, exercising regularly (any activity is good activity), not smoking (anything), and maintaining a normal weight (BMI 18-25). Other lifestyle interventions can be helpful including getting a proper amount of sleep (7-8 hours per night) and not having stress in your life (lol), just to name a few.

Human beings have a physical heart that, on average, weighs about two thirds of a pound and is roughly 2.5 by 3.5 by 5 inches in size. Wow...a lot smaller than I would have imagined. It is the pump that propels the life blood to all the tissues in the body. Amazing that such a small structure can have such an important assignment.

Terms:

In the NT Greek Bible, heart is usually the term *kardia* (sometimes spelled *cardia*). In the OT Hebrew scriptures, heart is usually *leb* (or *lebab*). In all of these biblical heart terms, the Bible writers may be referring to the anatomical flesh heart but are most often referring to the inner, invisible, soul-spirit heart.

Heart

How Does Cupid Fit In?

In popular culture, the heart is often viewed as the seat and source of emotions, something to be broken or to be in love with. The heart is a prominent symbol for Valentine's Day.

Since each human has a soul, which includes the body and has spirit potential (covered in-depth in earlier sections), I would now like to turn attention to how Scripture seems to address the heart.

Researching the word *heart* in the Bible has been fascinating. Trying to categorize the inner, invisible heart purely into either soul or spirit has proven fruitless. Often in Scripture, the heart is categorized as part of the soul—mind, will, and emotions—because of its close association with emotions and feelings. However, in modern translations as well as the original Greek and Hebrew, heart (*leb, kardia*) is often used interchangeably with mind, will, inner part, soul, thinking, conscience, knowledge, determination, reflection, memory; seat(s) of appetite, courage, emotions, and passion...and more. It seems as though, biblically speaking, the term *heart* was intended by the Bible writers (and, therefore, by God) to be an all-inclusive term for all that encompasses man's soul-spirit.

> ### Tidbit:
> In an earlier section on theology, I referred to the fact that man is a soul-body with spirit ability. The Hebrew words for soul and spirit show up early in the Genesis account of creation...God's *Spirit* in Genesis 1:2...and man's *soul* associated with God's breath in Genesis 2:7.
>
> ### Super Interesting Nerding-Out Tidbit:
> Even though the concept of man's spirit (*ruach*, breath) is used in the early Genesis account, it is not until much later in Genesis 41:8 that the Bible actually uses the term *spirit* in reference to a man, and that man was a godless Pharaoh: *"And it came to pass in the morning that his (Pharaoh's) spirit was troubled..."* This was after man's infection with sin in the garden, after Adam and Eve's spirits died. Interesting. Something to ponder.

Holy and Wholistic Health!

> **Dr. Clark Pearl:**
>
> It seems to me (not a theologian) the scriptural term *heart* is being used as the umbrella term that would include man being a soul-spirit or a spirit-soul (discussed previously). Said another way, if soul is *nephesh* and **spirit** is *ruach*, **heart** is man's **nephesh-ruach** (or **ruach-nephesh**); in the Greek, heart would be man's *psyche-pneuma* (or *pneuma-psyche*), the very inner part of man that separates man from other animals that possess souls. Sorry if this seems confusing, but stay with me on this. The potential health ramifications of this concept are immense.

Although the words *soul* and *spirit* appear early in Scripture, the term heart (*leb*) does not show up in the Bible until many years later in Genesis 6:5 (KJV) in a pre-flood reference, and then it was not in a good context: *"And God saw that the wickedness of man was great in the earth, and that every imagination of the thoughts of his heart was only evil continually."* Interesting that this verse speaks of the thoughts of the heart; modern western scientific rational thought does not ascribe "thinking" to the heart.

All of this fascinating discussion (to me anyway) on the scriptural concept of heart brings me to the culmination of where I am going with all this. And, to reach that pinnacle pearl, I will digress into another brief discussion that I plan to cover thoroughly in a later chapter...a discussion about the brain, mind, and thoughts.

> **Associated Tidbit:**
>
> The human heart contains neurons—nerves. The heart muscle might have as many as 40,000 neurons. One of the primary functions of nerves outside of the central nervous system throughout the body is detecting sensations...and feelings.

The thought (pardon the pun) I would like to bring out is that modern neuroscience seems to have reached a consensus that our anatomical brains made of neuron cells produce thoughts and that anatomical brain tissue can be changed over time, a concept called neuroplasticity. Many neuroscientists believe that our thought life...our specific thoughts...affect and change the structure and anatomy and function of the underlying brain tissue on which thoughts travel. Fascinating and paradigm-shifting!

Some have called the neurons in the heart the Intrinsic Cardiac Nervous System—ICNS for short. Neurons in the heart fall under the medical term cardiac neuroanatomy (I just wanted to mention that term to try and sound smart). One function of the ICNS is to help regulate heart

> ### What Stays in Vagus?
> The vagus nerve, also known as cranial nerve number 10, is responsible for supplying information back to the brain from the internal organs (heart, stomach, pancreas, liver, kidneys, etc.)... information our conscious minds might not always perceive. In other words, much unconscious information is constantly supplied back to the brain that keeps our bodies functioning normally. If we were aware of these continuous sensations (heart beating, lungs breathing, intestines squirming, etc.) at a conscious level, we would have a hard time functioning in daily life.
>
> ### The Heart Brain:
> Some have called the heart the third brain...the brain in the heart (the other two "brains" will be described in detail later). A brain in the heart with associated sensory feeling potential gives whole new meaning to phrases such as "I feel it in my heart."

rhythms and prevent abnormal heart racing or abnormal heart slowing... to help pace the heart. The neurons in the heart also supply information back to the brain through the vagus nerve.

Another digression—one day, I was outside exercising on my favorite nature trail. I was contemplating how thoughts can actually change the brain...pondering...and a related concept entered my heart (again, pardon the pun). If thoughts can change the brain, I wonder if it is possible for emotions to biologically affect, alter, and change the heart?

Holy and Wholistic Health!

> ### Tidbit:
> I already knew at least one documented way emotions can affect the heart. Takotsubo cardiomyopathy is a temporary heart condition (usually a pathologically enlarged heart) that can be triggered by serious physical illness or surgery but can also be triggered by stressful situations and extreme emotions...literally a broken heart brought on by a broken heart.
>
> ### Another Related Tidbit:
> Pathologically (diseased) enlarged hearts are a different process than the strengthening of the heart muscle that comes from regular cardio exercise. These are two anatomically and physiologically different processes. However, over-exercising (which most of us are in no danger of being accused of) can lead to unhealthy heart conditions. Quoting from the always reliable medical authority Wikipedia: "Overworking your heart causes the heart muscle to thicken, like any muscle being worked strenuously. Over time, this can lead to atrial fibrillation, and to heart failure."

The Bible refers to changing the brain by changing the thoughts as the renewing of the mind: *"...be transformed by the renewing of your mind"* (Romans 12:2). Renewing the mind involves intentionally thinking the good and healthy thoughts of God on a regular basis.

Now shift back to the heart—"be heart transformed by the renewing of your emotions" (a Dr. Clark version of Romans 12:2). Said differently—is it possible that experiencing the good and healthy emotions of God on a regular basis might affect and change the anatomy and physiology of my heart cells? Is it possible that I can renew, heal, restore, cure, and repair my heart by regularly experiencing God's healthy emotions?

> ### Spiritual Tidbit:
> Spiritually, a hard heart can be softened and made pliable and restored by forgiving and loving. The blood of Jesus sprinkled (applied) to a hard heart will begin a change of heart (biblical repentance) and can take a hard heart and make it soft.

This concept is mostly intuitive and (maybe a little) scientific.

Heart

> **OT Echoes:**
> *"I will give you a new heart and put a new spirit within you; and I will take the heart of stone out of your flesh and give you a heart of flesh"* (Ezekiel 36:26).

To elaborate negatively, the term hard-hearted is commonly used when someone has put up emotional walls over their heart and emotions. They have developed a callous heart. Hard-heartedness is mentioned throughout the entirety of the Bible when an individual becomes callous against God and people. Hard-heartedness is a serious spiritual condition that may... probably...eventually maybe...produce a real, physical hard heart—think heart attack, heart damage, arteriosclerosis (hardening of the arteries).

Keep It Soft

When I am worshiping at home, I like to sing the song "Soften My Heart" by Cindy Gough. It speaks of keeping my heart pliable and soft by regularly spending time with the Lord and allowing my tears to tenderize my heart.

Hardness is easy; softness takes work. Insensitivity is easy; sensitivity takes work. And time.

Fresh Fruit

I see a correlation between a soft heart and fresh, ripe fruit...and a correlation with a healthy relationship, especially a marriage relationship. I

> **Covid Correlation:**
> I am writing this paragraph as my wife and I are on the third day of "isolation" due to being Covid positive. We are now physically doing fine; we experienced just a little touch of mild flu symptoms for the first few days. However, just the change in routine and the actual health symptoms made it easier for me to be insensitive toward my wife, the one I love. I am now changing this. The love of God along with the help of Jesus and the Holy Spirit are helping me to change this.

> **Covid Correlation #2:**
> The Covid pandemic has not just produced health-related disease and death. It also created major financial, employment, social, and political upheaval—like waves of disruptions and uncertainty continually pounding against a shoreline. The Covid era disruptions have made it very easy, almost natural, for many to become hard-hearted and insensitive toward others.

think most would agree that a healthy, intimate marriage and fresh fruit and a soft heart are good and valuable things. Yet all of these take time and energy and can be easily lost if not continually receiving intentional care and input.

Warm It Up

Fruit can spoil very quickly, a warm marriage relationship can become cold and apathetic, a soft heart toward the Lord and others can easily develop calluses unintentionally over time. Without continual attention and input, fruit spoils, relationships grow cold, and intimacy with the Lord is easily lost or turns into religious rituals.

On the positive side, there has been much research on the effects of positive emotions such as laughter, joy, happiness, love, peace...and the positive health benefits these emotions can produce. Intui-

> **Mega Pearl:**
> Developing hardness and insensitivity is the natural order of things, like the entropy law of physics which states all things are moving toward chaos and disorder without continual energy expenditure. Maintaining softness and sensitivity to the Lord and people is vital; it is crucial. This is the big one. Getting this right may be the most important thing a person does for their overall health; maintaining a soft heart helps me understand purpose and meaning in life. I keep my heart soft by regularly being with the Lord, guarding my heart with all diligence for out of it spring the issues of life. *"Guard your heart with all diligence for out of it spring the issues of life."*

Heart

> **Fun Verse:**
> *"A joyful heart is good medicine..."* (Proverbs 17:22 NASB). Another translation says, *"a joyful, cheerful heart brings healing to both body and soul"* (aha!); another says, *"if you are cheerful, you feel good,"* and another says, *"a happy heart is good medicine and a joyful mind causes healing,"* and another addresses overall attitude by saying, *"a cheerful disposition is good for your health."*

tively this makes sense. Science is starting to make some headway into how positive emotions and experiences may benefit health.

Can I Do My Own Heart Surgery?

If an individual is going to renew his/her emotions to experience the emotions of God, they must ask, "What are God's emotions?" Galatians 5:22-23 talks about the fruit (plural) of the Spirit—God's emotions and qualities through His Holy Spirit—love, joy, peace, patience, kindness, goodness, gentleness, faithfulness, self-control. There are other biblical

> **Tidbit:**
> Obviously, emotions and thoughts are intertwined. For explanation and understanding purposes, we often separate them; this helps when focusing on either aspect to make a point. But experiencing emotions involves thoughts, and thinking involves emotions. Perhaps this is why the biblical term *heart* is translated in some instances as mind and other times refers to emotions.
>
> **Heart Murmur Pearl:**
> A heart murmur is defined as an abnormal sound that can be heard when listening to the heart with a stethoscope; it is caused by a structural or functional abnormality of the biological heart. The obvious soul parallel—when a person is murmuring with their words, there is an obvious abnormality of their inner heart.

> **Pearl:**
> My late friend/mentor/pastor had an interesting saying. He said if there was no afterlife, following Jesus and keeping His commandments was still the best, happiest, most rewarding, most fulfilling lifestyle possible. I agree. After trying many other pathways...through the school of hard knocks...by trial and error...by lots of errors...I agree truly following Jesus is the most fulfilling, rewarding, and healthiest life possible!

examples of God's emotions that humans might experience by being with God, by being in His presence, by having a relationship with Him...but the list from Galatians is a good place to start.

Here's a big health pearl: If I continually and ongoingly experience the emotions of God in my heart—in both my natural, anatomical heart (*leb, kardia*) and in my invisible, soul-spirit heart (*nephesh-ruach, psyche-pneuma*)—is it possible that those emotions of God might change, heal, and soften my biological heart...similar to how healthy thoughts change the structure of the brain? Said another way, can I do my own heart surgery on a daily basis by continually experiencing the emotions of God—by renewing my emotions to the emotions of God? What an amazing thought!

I remember exactly where I was on my favorite nature trail when this thought entered my mind and my heart. I got excited. Renewing my emotions to be the emotions of God is a truly wholistic, safe, organic, health habit to benefit my heart! And, if science never confirms this possible theory as being accurate, I know God's emotions will still benefit my spirit-soul-body—and benefit those around me (my family, friends, acquaintances, and society in general).

Tears and a Broken Heart

I have a question. Why is it our eyes leak fluid when we are experiencing pain or sadness or grief...or even when we are extremely happy? Why is the body's response to these different stimuli crying tears? I have often pondered this but will admit I don't ultimately know why God wired us this way.

Some of the reasons speculated by others for why we cry when experiencing soul extremes or physical pain are interesting. One thought is that tears—which come from the lacrimal sac at the outer-upper corner of the eye and flow across our eyeballs before draining into the nasolacrimal duct at the inner corner of the eye and into the nasal passages—contain and release feel good chemicals...prolactin...endorphins...enkephalin...in essence, crying is a form of self-soothing. Seems reasonable.

Tear Tidbits:

The Greek word for tear is *dakry*. An infection of a tear sac, lacrimal sac, is called *dacryocystitis*. The Latin for tear is *lacrimam*. Crying is also called *lacrimation*.

Paul's Tears:

The Bible records that the Apostle Paul, one of the great Bible writers, fathers, and church-planting missionaries of the New Testament, felt such anguish of soul when he was providing loving correction to one of his young church groups that he was brought to tears (2 Corinthians 2:4). If someone feels led to bring loving correction into my life, I hope they have tears in their eyes—tears of brokenness and humility.

Along this same line of thought, a distinction is made between what are called psychic tears (such as emotional pain tears) and reflexive tears (such as when peeling an onion). It is believed that psychic tears have higher levels of the feel-good chemicals than reflexive tears.

Incidentally, healthy grieving is called a lament in the Bible. Proper, God-designed, healthy grieving is good for your health...soothing the soul...helping the heart-soul-spirit heal after experiencing loss or deep soul pain.

David's Tears:

In the OT, David was often in anguish of soul in his early years. For many years, he regularly had a murderous madman (King Saul) chasing him, trying to take him out. He often wrote songs from deep sorrow (the Psalms) and in one place said of God: *"You keep track of all my sorrows. You have collected all my tears in your bottle..."* (Psalm 56:8 NLT). Geek note: the Hebrew OT word for tears is *dima'h*.

Holy and Wholistic Health!

Having a healthy, physical heart—and a healthy soul-spirit heart—will produce energy and vitality and an overall sense of well-being, and this in turn helps an individual stay free of disease, both now and hopefully many years to come! (Note: Some of this same material on tears will be discussed further in a later section under "Beyond" entitled "When Life Leaks.")

Blood Pressure

"The Flow of Life"

Closely associated with the heart, the pump of life, are the physical forces that are experienced in the heart and the arteries. These forces are known as the blood pressure.

Physiology class was fascinating. In physiology class, I witnessed for the first time a beating heart. Usually an animal. Later, in anatomy class, I was able to dissect a human heart...but...for obvious reasons, that heart was not beating. The living, beating heart of physiology demonstrated up close how this blob of muscular tissue actually beats by a muscular contraction starting in one area and then progressively contracting in a wave throughout the entirety of the heart. The progressive contracting wave of a beating heart reminded me of how a wet cloth is wrung out in a twisted, squeezing motion.

Once the heart beats—squeezing in on itself forcefully—by contracting its muscle layers, the rush of blood is pumped out of the heart into the aorta, which eventually branches like a tree into smaller and smaller arteries that feed all bodily tissues. At least that's where the left-sided heart chambers pump blood into. The other side, the right chambers, pump blood into a vessel that goes to the lungs...but that's another story.

I am a simple-minded fellow, and my brain works best by simple illustrations. Regarding blood pressure, the top blood pressure number is the systolic blood pressure which is the measure of pressure inside the heart and arteries at its maximum pressure. Maximum pressure is immediately

> **Tidbit:**
> If the lowest pressure in the heart were 0, the person would be—you guessed it—dead. No pressure, no flow, no life.
>
> **Rabbit Trail Tidbit:**
> All living things require pressure and tension and movement. Pressure in life, otherwise known as stress, is normal and necessary for living systems to function. A life without pressure...without stress...is no life at all.

during and after the heart beats. Makes sense.

The lower blood pressure number, the diastolic blood pressure, is the pressure inside the heart and arteries when the blood pressure is at its lowest. The lowest pressure in the heart is immediately before the heart beats. So far so good.

From the moment the heart muscle finishes contracting, releasing its tension, until the moment immediately before the heart contracts again is the time the heart muscle gets its relative rest. This segment of time is called diastole.

Unlike skeletal muscles, such as the biceps muscle, which require time to recuperate and rebuild in between workouts, the heart muscle only gets its rest in the brief period called diastole. Diastole, the time the heart gets to rest, lasts about 0.5 second.

The fancy medical term for high blood pressure is hypertension. High blood pressure is diagnosed when either the top systolic pressure or the bottom diastolic pressure or both are higher than normal. Many things

> **Rest Pressures:**
> Even during necessary sleep, the human body is never completely at rest. Biochemical reactions are always happening. Physiological processes are occurring. Energy is being expended at the cellular level, albeit overall energy expenditure is less than when awake; this total body energy expenditure at rest is known as the resting metabolic rate. Blood is still flowing. The heart is still beating. Lungs are still breathing. Intestines are still squirming. The blood pressure and heart rate do normally dial down to lower levels during sleep.

Fun Potential Spiritual Correlate:

Since systolic high BP is when the heart is "working" too hard at too high of a pressure, I have wondered about when stress contributes to high blood pressure. Might there be a correlation between when a person is overworking—such as when one is labeled a workaholic—and the top systolic blood pressure rising?

Obvious Associated Potential Correlation:

Since diastolic high BP is when the heart BP is too high "at rest," might there be a correlation between when a person is not adequately resting—not sleeping well, not psychologically or internally or mentally resting—and the diastolic blood pressure being too high?

My Personal Experience:

I regularly check my BP and seem to have found correlations between times of high systolic BP when I am overworking. I also seem to have found times of elevated diastolic BP when I am not resting well—usually when not psychologically resting well (when I feel stressed). I will continue to check out this hypothesis on myself over time. I am sure many other correlations might be found regarding elevated systolic and diastolic BP readings.

can contribute to high blood pressure, one of which is ingesting too much salt or sodium.

Blood Pressure and Circulation

Similar to heart disease developing by plaque buildup and blockage of heart arteries, plaque can also accumulate in any artery of the body. Plaque deposits in the peripheral arteries outside the heart are termed atherosclerotic peripheral vascular disease—ASPVD for short. Other terms for this include peripheral arterial disease (PAD) and peripheral vascular disease (PVD).

Holy and Wholistic Health!

> **Circulation Tidbit:**
> When a person says, "My circulation is not good," one of the ways this might be manifested is if flow of blood to the legs is insufficient because of a totally or partially blocked artery in or to the legs. Arteries are not the only blood vessels to potentially develop problems; blocked or damaged veins are another form of poor circulation.

High blood pressure has been implicated as one of the contributing factors to both heart disease and peripheral vascular disease. Blocked peripheral arteries in the brain can lead to a stroke. (Strokes will be discussed in a later section.) Diminished blood flow to any bodily organ peripherally (such as diminished blood flow to a kidney artery) will result in tissue damage or tissue death (in this case kidney damage or kidney death).

Blockage-type plaque buildup evolving over time is one danger of elevated blood pressure. Another immediate danger of high blood pressure, which seems more intuitive, is if the high pressure finds a weak spot in an artery or vein. If the weak spot forms a pouch...a little balloon so-to-speak... it is called an aneurysm. In these situations, the weak, damaged vessel might break and cause a stroke or heart attack or aortic rupture...none of which are good. High blood pressure is also considered a risk factor for developing other serious conditions such as kidney failure and dementia.

> **Pearl:**
> It has been reported that many pleasurable things which produce joy and happiness—such as listening to music, laughing, spending time in nature, dancing, exercising (if that sort of thing brings you pleasure), healthy social connections, healthy marriages, beloved pets, and many other pleasurable things—can lower blood pressure. I have found this to be true in my own body as I regularly use Dr. Jonny as a guinea pig for many self-experiments, such as monitoring my blood pressure in many different situations and at different times of the day and night.

Blood Pressure

> ### Corollary Pearl:
> I have seen many times in my medical practice where negative emotions or unpleasant experiences have increased a person's blood pressure when their BP was previously normal. Intuitive. And dangerous. I remember one person developing a stroke-level high blood pressure seemingly overnight that was not controlled on four different blood pressure-lowering medications. One day they came to my office and their blood pressure was normal, and they were not taking any medications. I asked what was different? They said they quit their job and got a new job (in this case, they said it was a toxic relationship at work that they had to get away from).
>
> ### Another Corollary Pearl:
> The biblical concept of the sabbath is the practice of taking one day off work per week. No work for one day...and in its place spending time with family, friends...perhaps with spiritual relationships...worshiping...relaxing...doing the enjoyable things that you might not have time to do the other six days. Rather than a religious legalistic ritual (listed as one of the Ten Commandments given to Moses in the Old Testament), the weekly sabbath rest is a brilliant potentially heart-healthy, blood pressure-lowering, and mentally healthy and relational healthy habit!

Blood pressure is an interesting and paradoxical thing. If the blood pressure is too high, you have trouble. If it is too low, it's not good (dizziness, fainting, weakness). If there is no blood pressure, you're dead.

It is actually good for the heart to be regularly stressed in a healthy way, otherwise known as cardio exercise. Exercise makes the heart temporarily work harder...beat faster, more vigorously—thereby causing an increase in heart rate and blood pressure. A heart that is not periodically stressed in a healthy way can become architecturally weak and reactively sluggish; "soft in an unhealthy way" would be one way to describe it. The heart and blood pressure that are regularly stressed by proper exercise and allowed to recover should become strong, healthy...able to respond to life's stressors in a healthy way.

Pearl:

Exercise is HUGE when it comes to helping control blood pressure. Regular exercise has the effect of lowering blood pressure slowly, progressively. Mix that slow, beneficial effect with the fact that a good bout of exercise lowers BP immediately after the work-out.

Example:

I had a patient many years ago who would come in for her regular BP medication visit. She would walk three miles immediately before the visit because she knew that her blood pressure would always be very good, even better than usual, at her check-up because she had just exercised. Kind of like when as a kid, I would brush my teeth for three hours right before a dental visit...hoping that would take care of the fact that I hadn't taken care of my teeth appropriately since the last visit. I was hoping I could brush away any cavities. It didn't work. I had lots of cavities as a kid.

A healthy heart needs to be able to respond to life's stressors in a healthy way. For instance, when a person stands up from the sitting position, there should be an immediate, temporary rise in blood pressure to accommodate for gravity's effects to maintain adequate blood flow to the brain, thereby not passing out. Healthy, reactive blood pressure should then level out back down to a normal pressure.

Does this Doughnut Make Me Look Fat?

I thought it appropriate to discuss fat in the context of heart and blood pressure, as being overweight or even obese is considered a risk factor for many metabolic conditions such as heart disease, high blood pressure, diabetes, stroke, degenerative arthritis, and different forms of dementia (just to name a few).

The healthcare community uses many parameters to classify if someone is overweight—actual scale weight, waist circumference, waist-to-hip ratio, actual body fat percentage calculations, and BMI (and other pa-

> **BMI Tidbits:**
>
> BMI, otherwise known as body mass index, is derived by looking at a person's height and weight. A BMI of 18.5-25 is considered in the normal range. If a BMI is less than 18.5, it falls within the underweight range; a BMI of 25-30 is considered overweight; 30 or higher is considered obese. BMI calculators can be easily found online with a Google search.

rameters). BMI is probably the parameter that is currently used the most in traditional healthcare settings.

Interestingly, a few research studies in recent years seem to indicate it might be healthier for a person to be in the upper range of normal BMI as compared to the lower end of BMI range. One speculation was that if a person had a little extra padding (a slightly higher BMI) and developed a serious condition, they might be able to overcome the crisis condition easier. I hope this is true since I have tended to be in the higher ranges of BMI most of my life. However, this will certainly need more research to determine whether there might be any fact to this. For now, BMI 18.5-25 is considered normal.

Fat a Blessing?

Interestingly, the OT biblical writers considered fat to be a blessing, a sign of abundance and prosperity. Makes sense. We have such a problem with being overweight in our culture because we have such an overabundance of blessing (food), and we (I) tend to overeat. "All things in moderation"

> **OT Echoes:**
>
> In the OT Hebrew scriptures, ingesting fat (and blood) was ceremonially strictly forbidden: *"This shall be a perpetual statute throughout your generations in all your dwellings: you shall eat neither fat nor blood"* (Leviticus 3:17). The fat of a sacrificial animal's viscera and organs were to be removed on the altar when making a sacrifice to the Lord; the animal fat was to be burned to the Lord as a holy sacrifice, a sweet-smelling aroma ceremonially to God (Leviticus 3:14-16). Fat and blood were considered holy, sacred, pure…reserved for God alone.

Holy and Wholistic Health!

> **Reference Verse Before the Flood:**
>
> *"And God said, 'See, I have given you every herb that yields seed which is on the face of all the earth, and every tree whose fruit yields seed; to you it shall be for food'"* (Genesis 1:29).
>
> **Reference Verse After the Flood:**
>
> *"...every beast of the earth, on every bird of the air, on all that move on the earth, and on all the fish of the sea. They are given into your hand. Every moving thing that lives shall be food for you. I have given you all things, even as the green herbs. But you shall not eat flesh with its life, that is, its blood"* (Genesis 9:2-4).

is a good health and life slogan. And, you don't just have to eat fat to get fat; our bodies have wonderful metabolic capabilities to turn overindulgence in carbohydrates and proteins into fat storage (that was a sarcastic facetious statement if you didn't pick up on it).

This brings up an entire topic that is interesting and somewhat controversial. Long story short—when the people in the OT started eating animals for food, which was ceremonially allowed after Noah and the flood, the lifespan of humans began to go down. Previously, when they were only eating a plant-based diet (vegan), the lifespan of humans was extremely long, often from around 600-900 years.

I have heard the explanation that the diminishing lifespan after the flood was just a result of sin entering the world and spreading; its effects of death and disease were finally having enough time to affect lifespan. I believe there is truth in that statement. However, I find it interesting that there is a coincidence with the fact that mankind was, after the flood, ceremonially allowed to eat animals and animal products...meat, eggs, milk, cheese, etc. Vegan to non-vegan. And the lifespan started to decrease simultaneously, catching up with the prediction...declaration...prophecy made by God in Genesis 6:3 where He said, *"My Spirit shall not strive with man forever, for he is indeed flesh; yet his days shall be one hundred and twenty years."* Many years later, Moses lived to be 120.

Blood Pressure

> ### Interesting Personal Correlation:
>
> For over five years, I have experimented with different forms of fasting for health and religious purposes. I have actually written a short book about my experience with intermittent fasting. One thing I have noticed consistently and repeatedly when I do a vegan fast—biblically speaking, a Daniel Fast of no meat or animal products—I will lose weight, which is expected. However, additionally my cholesterol levels go from good to great, as if I am taking a cholesterol-lowering medication such as Lipitor...getting the benefits without any medication side effects. High or abnormal cholesterol levels and being overweight are significant risk factors for heart disease, stroke, and circulation problems and can affect other metabolic disease processes such as diabetes, high blood pressure, and dementia processes.

When I am eating vegan only, I will eat a significant amount of plant fats, usually in the form of avocados and olives and nuts. These high levels of plant fat intake do not negatively affect my weight or my cholesterol levels; on the contrary, they are both benefitted. When I start to add any cheese or milk or meat, my cholesterol numbers shift away from being stellar. Interestingly, when I added eggs to my vegan eating, I did not see the negative cholesterol shift. This was a one-time experiment for me; I intend to check that again on myself in the future.

> ### The Fat Soul:
>
> *"...Let your soul delight itself in fatness"* (Isaiah 55:2 KJV).

Olives, Olive Oil, and Fatness

Olives are abundant in the Mediterranean Sea area, the region in which all of the Bible is set. I like olives, well, at least most kinds of olives. Olives can be pressed and the resultant drippings collected—olive oil. Most modern health groups believe olive oil has positive health benefits and should be used instead of most of the other plant oils that are available, whether in cooking or used as a topping garnishment as when used as a salad dressing.

Holy and Wholistic Health!

Here's the thing about olives. Olives and olive oil are high in fat, but olive fat is a plant fat and not animal fat. Other examples of high-fat plants (non-animal) are avocados and nuts. More and more research studies are

Personal tidbit:

When I do my annual January Daniel Fast, a vegan fast, my intake percentage will have a high quantity of olives, avocados, nuts, and other high-fat plants. My metabolic numbers including blood sugar, cholesterol, blood pressure, and weight all respond favorably (elaborated on in my booklet called *Waiting to Eat*). When I start eating animal products and animal fat again (meat, butter, cheese, dairy, etc.), my metabolic numbers are not as stellar.

OT Echoes:

In the OT, olives and olive oil were often symbolically and practically considered to be evidence of fatness, prosperity, abundance, and blessing. Fat and oil were often interchangeable terms. The infamous Psalm 23 has a phrase in verse five: *"...you honor me by anointing my head with oil. My cup overflows with blessings..."* (NLT version). Many other OT verses reflect similar blessings associated with the oil.

Interesting Tidbit?

The OT Hebrew word for oil is pronounced *sheh'-men*; the Blue Letter Bible mentions that this fatty oil was even used as a medicament (fancy word) health treatment often in the form of an unguent (another fancy word), meaning as a soft greasy or viscous substance used as an ointment or for lubrication.

OT Tabernacle Echoes:

In the OT, the ever-merciful God invented a way for His people to interact and have a relationship with Him, which was His strong desire. The problem: God's holy and beautiful and pure nature prevented non-holy people from approaching and interacting with Him. His solution: The OT tabernacle. In brief, the tabernacle had an outer court where there was a place for water and animal blood sacrifice cleansing. Entering further in was an

(Cont): inner place, the Holy Place, a place where only priests could go; the Holy Place had a table for special bread, a lampstand in which oil was burned for light, and the altar of incense where sweet-smelling fragrant incense sacrifices were continually offered to the Lord. Beyond this was the innermost place, the Holy of Holies, containing the ark of the covenant, representing God's presence and His dwelling place. In the OT before Jesus, the tabernacle format was how people approached and had relationship with the pure and beautiful Father God. In the NT, after Christ sacrificed His blood for all mankind to have relationship with God, the outer court became obsolete (sacrifices and cleansing continually available in and through Jesus), and the veil between the Holy Place and the Holy of Holies was destroyed. In the presence of Christ (the bread, the Word) and the Holy Spirit (the flow of the oil of anointing with light and power), relationship with the all-merciful and beautiful Father was re-established!

More Tabernacle Echoes:

Many different applications and parallel examples can and have been drawn from the tabernacle imagery and reality. For good health, I would like to mention the parallels of the OT outer court (body) and inner court (soul) and innermost Holy of Holies (Spirit). Before Christ, all that was possible was soul-body life (with spirit receptors and brief Spirit encounters). After Christ, the soul-body could now become spirit-soul-body again...the bread (Christ) and the flow of oil (Holy Spirit) constantly at work in the realm of the soul...on the earth...benefitting the body and uniting the soul back to God's Spirit Life as an ongoing, vital reality. Spirit-soul-body health at it's finest...now and hopefully for many years to come!

claiming the positive health benefit of plant fats, especially in contrast with animal fats.

A healthy heart with healthy blood pressure and healthy cholesterol levels and a healthy weight and healthy body fat percentages will maximize energy, vitality, and well-being, helping to prevent disease and hopefully live a long life. *"Keep your heart with all diligence, for out of it spring the issues of life"* (Proverbs 4:23).

Fun Break

Nerding out on God

I'm writing this passage in the dead of winter...literally. It was 10 below zero two days ago; I believe that was a record low for us. It has been snowing off and on for about five days with lingering accumulation on the roads. This is very unusual, not typical for southwest Missouri. Two days ago, I was at the medical office getting ready for the day and...boom! The power went out. We had the privilege of experiencing our first rolling blackout, previously planned by the utility company to preserve energy for the region. I know people in chillier parts of the country laugh at us for making a big deal out of these things, but this is a big deal for us. Incidentally, earlier this week Austin, Texas, had a lower temperature as a daily high than Anchorage, Alaska, has had all winter. I saw real hockey players playing real hockey on our iced-over community pond. We just don't see such things here.

I was walking and praying last weekend on our frozen tundra (my exaggeration) and came to the edge of a frozen lake. I was spacing-out as I gazed across the icy landscape. I saw a straight line on the ice lake... no animal or human footprints around the line (I could see all of the other animal footprints in the snow that had ventured out on the lake). As I studied it closer, it became apparent the line was actually a breaking point, a fault line, where the ice was starting to thaw...almost like two plates of ice contacting one another.

Pondering and enjoying my walk, I walked around to another vantage point and saw where the fault line eventually stopped at an already thawed circle of water. The very cold water in the small puddle—and under the ice plates—was moving, flowing. I continued to look and pray, think and ponder. The frigid wind blew the top of the chilly water. Two flows, one at the top of the water and one under the ice.

Back to the Beginning

I thought of Genesis 1:2 (NASB): *"...the Spirit of God was moving (hovering) over the surface of the waters."* Review: *Spirit* in Hebrew OT is *ruach*, which translates as **wind** or breath or air. God was literally blowing His wind-air-breath-Spirit over the surface of the waters.

I thought of Genesis 1:6 (NLT): *"Then God said, 'Let there be a **space** (Hebrew raqiya') between the waters of the heavens from the waters of the earth.'"* Waters of the heavens that flow...wind, Spirit, breath, air...oxygen. Waters of the earth...water. The flow of heaven intersects the flow of earth at the space, the *raqiya'*...Bible translators translate the term *raqiya'* as firmament, vault, space, expanses. The original Hebrew also defines *raqiya'* with the words surface (solid), base, support. Stay with me...I'm going somewhere with all this nerding out stuff.

Continuing on, Genesis 1:7-8: *"And God made the raqiya', and divided the waters which were under the raqiya' from the waters which were above the raqiya': and it was so. And God called the raqiya' Heaven..."* The Hebrew word used here for Heaven is *shamayim* and is translated as visible heavens, atmosphere, sky, visible universe. Having fun yet?

And then, Genesis 1:9-10 (KJV): *"And God said, 'Let the waters under the heaven be gathered together unto one place, and let the dry land appear: and it was so. And God called the dry land Earth; and the gathering together of the waters called he Seas: and God saw that it was good.'"* Did I previously mention that I love the early chapters of Genesis?

I am not a Hebrew scholar or an educated Bible interpreter, but I do know translating from one language to another can be difficult, due to the differences in culture and worldview and nuances in word usage. Also, the number of words available in one language may be vastly different than the number of words in another language. Such seems to be the case in Genesis 1:10 with the phrase *"the dry land Earth."* The original language interpreters note that the term "the dry" is *yabbashah* (dry land, dry ground) and the second part of the phrase—"land earth"—is being translated as the Hebrew *'erets*—defined as land, earth, piece of ground, surface of the earth, soil. By far and away, the Hebrew OT mostly uses *'erets* in the context of land or earth.

Pearl:
As I gazed at the winter wonderland in front of me, I realized the flow of God's heaven (oxygen air) and the flow of earth (inorganic water)—at the point where the flows of heaven and earth meet—is where God created life... and humanity. Invisible became visible. And, it is no surprise that the visible life forms, humans in particular, would be a creature of flow...of oxygen and water...of blood (*'erets* life). The meeting of heaven and earth is where God's good pleasure for physical life exists.

Pearl Said Another Way:
Humans, as spirit-souls (or even as soul-spirits,) thrive best at the intersection of heaven and earth; they thrive spiritually, mentally, emotionally, relationally, and physically in bodies—at the intersection of heaven's flows and earth's flows. This was God's design from the beginning; even in the new creation resurrection life of NT Jesus believers, the Bible reveals Jesus and resurrected individuals to have a body, it is just changed into a different body from what it was prior. A soul needs a body.

Enough Nerding Out Already

The meeting of heaven and earth, the fault line between the flows, is solid. This solid earth produces the plants and the animals...the **bread** that mixes with the breath in the blood of life. This was and is God's good pleasure!

If the physical earth—which itself has a flow—becomes too dry, not getting rain from the heavens, it becomes hard, it gets crusty, easily cracked. If the earth becomes too cold, the flowing water solidifies and becomes hard. Things that are too hard, including the earth and the ice and the human heart (physical and spiritual hard-heartedness), will eventually break...thaw...crack...at the weak points, the fault lines; when the hardness cracks open, the encased flow that has been underneath can spring out.

It's All About Flow

Good health is the **flow** of energy and strength and vitality, absent of disease and dysfunction, producing maximum well-being now and for many years to come.

Let's now turn to the bread.

BREAD

Stomach and Intestines
"The Bread of Life"

Humans are fearfully and wonderfully made (Psalm 139). To me, one of the quirkiest parts of our make-up is our digestive system. The digestive system—the mouth, esophagus, stomach, intestines, colon, and beyond (wink)—is one big, long tube...also known as the alimentary canal...the tube from stem to stern...from mouth to, well..."uranus" (so sorry about that). The digestive tract is reported to be up to 30 feet in length in adults.

Many classify all parts of the digestive system as actually outside of the body since both ends have openings to the outside world. As a result, many bacteria and germs colonize the GI tract and are a normal part of our lives. Some gut bacteria are harmful when they multiply and grow, becoming parasitic and resulting in problems. Helicobacter Pylori leads to ulcers; the Clostridium Difficile bacteria leads to colitis; and the parasite Giardia causes much intestinal distress. Other germs seem to have a healthy, even symbiotic benefit to our health. This has led to the large and expanding branch of research on healthy gut germs (gut flora), resulting in helpful interventions such as probiotics and other treatment approaches...even fecal transplants (I'm not gonna touch that one with a ten-foot pole; insert

> **Interesting Correlation:**
> Some bacteria in the colon will ferment any fermentable foodstuffs that pass from the small intestine into the large intestine. Fermentation produces some usable energy and some by-product chemicals...and gas...multiple types of gas. That's all I'm gonna say about that.

Sauerkraut Anyone?
Many proponents of the healthy gut microbiome theory believe certain fermented foods promote healthy gut bacteria—foods such as sauerkraut, kimchi, yogurt...maybe even the popular drink Kombucha.

Worms? Really?
In my modern medical practice, I rarely see patients who have infestations of intestinal worms. The most common worm that I see is the small pinworm, the most common worm infection in the US, more common in kids and those in crowded, poor-hygienic situations. I will not describe how the "scotch-tape test" will diagnose it, but (pun, sorry) will just mention how easy it is to treat with a medication once identified. In all my years, I have only once seen a roundworm infection...a larger worm like an earthworm or fishing worm...which can be contracted by eating poorly cooked meat or by indiscriminately eating various things from the yard or soil. Enuf said.

surprised emoji face here). I will defer to the expertise and knowledge of others regarding this growing segment of GI health science called the gut microbiome and related concepts such as leaky gut syndrome.

Gross Tidbits:
Many of the scientific formal terms relating to the digestive tract are gross-sounding words. I may, for the sake of fun junior high humor, mention some of these along the way. For instance, mastication is the proper term for chewing. I remember being on a family vacation road trip and, to pass the time, we tried to recall as many fancy, yucky, gross medical terms as possible, most of which related to digestion.

It seems as though the main purpose of the human alimentary canal is to process and digest our food; food I will collectively refer to as "bread." When any bread (food or liquid) enters the mouth, it immediately starts to be broken down...pulverized...processed physically and chemically into its basic constituents such as protein, fat, carbohydrates, water, minerals, and vitamins.

As the pulverized foodstuffs pass from the mouth into the esopha-

Stomach and Intestines

gus, the blob of emulsified nutrition is called chyme. This blob continues to be further refined and broken down... from the stomach's acidic juices into the small intestine's digestive enzymes into the colon, otherwise known as the large intestine. The colon is essentially the final processing facility. By the time the gross blob of foodstuff reaches the final part of the colon, almost all nutrition and water—the good stuff—has been absorbed across the lining of the digestive tube and into the bloodstream. The remaining "blob o' stuff" is no longer valuable to the body and is released back to the outside world from which it came.

> **Other Fun Words and Definitions:**
>
> Swallowing is deglutition; burping is eructation; borborygmus is when the stomach is growling. One phrase that especially caught my attention was the gastro-colic reflex, which is when a person may get a signal that they have to have a BM after eating food (or drinking coffee).

In the earlier sections, I alluded to the fact "bread" (our nutrition in all its forms) is one of the key components that come from the outside world and ends up in our blood as a key component for life (along with oxygen, the "breath," and the inorganic "water of life"). Bread and breath in the blood. The bread comes from God's living organic world at the interface of heaven (air, oxygen, spirit) and earth (water and other minerals and nutrients). Reviewing the spiritual implications, this strongly resembles and parallels how our souls (*nephesh*) are intricately intertwined with our bodies...and that our nephesh souls have spiritual potential, the ultimate goal of being a spirit-soul body. Humans are at the intersection of heaven and earth...the design of life and health from the beginning.

A Jack of Many Trades

As we humans try to study, understand, and make sense of our bodies, it seems as though the specialized tissue cells (such as brain, bone, GI tract) have a primary function, a primary role to play for healthy human functioning. The GI tract, for instance, seems to have as its main assignment to extract nutrition from the foodstuffs that we ingest. Clear. Simple. Focused. As we explore human anatomy and physiology, we find most specialized cells and specialized tissue making up specialized organs have at least one (if not many) secondary purpose to fulfill.

The Second Brain?

In the case of the GI tract, there is an extensive network of neurons (brain-type cells) in the gut lining, some estimates as high as 500 million neurons in the gut. This has been dubbed the enteric nervous system, enteric defined as relating to the intestines. This "brain in the gut" has been implicated in affecting not only digestion and nutrition but also moods and health...even the way a person thinks. The science concerning the digestive system is so very complex. The gut flora (otherwise known as the microbiome), combined with the "brain in the gut" enteric nervous system, affects all of our health and our thoughts, feelings, and actions—our souls. In other words, the gut plays a role in our overall health. An upset tummy may not just cause irritation and discomfort but may ruin your whole day.

A Personal Story

When I was in high school, I began to experience severe and sharp pains in my belly...belly being one of my favorite slang terms to include the stomach, abdomen, and lower GI tract. I loudly yelled to my friend, "Take me to the ER immediately...I can't stand the pain!" As we raced toward the hospital—he owned a Chevelle in the early 1980s and was going to drive fast anyway—a surprising thing happened. The pain stopped. It was gone. That stomach pain resolved.

A few years later, I had a similar flare-up of the same sharp abdominal pains. These pains continued off and on over the next few days...often worse after I would eat, and especially worse if I ate fatty, greasy, fried, spicy foods...my normal diet at the time. The pains would often feel like waves of sharp, stabbing pains. I went to see a clinic doctor, and he told me I had a spastic colon. I later learned the proper name for spastic colon is Irritable Bowel Syndrome, IBS for short.

Stomach and Intestines

> **Important Tidbit:**
> When using the abbreviated acronym IBS, it is crucial to distinguish which IBS is being referred to. IBS can, and often does, indicate my abnormal, painful muscular gut contractions, otherwise known as spastic colon (Irritable Bowel Syndrome). However, IBS can also be used when referring to Inflammatory Bowel Disease, a more serious group of GI problems that include Crohn's disease and Ulcerative Colitis.

The doctor gave me some pills—muscle relaxers for my abnormal intestinal muscle contractions—which helped a little. He told me to change my diet away from fast food and processed foods and eat a healthier, bland diet. I was in college at the time and too lazy to make my lunch so I would often eat out. The only eating establishment I found where I could eat the healthier, bland diet was the Heritage Cafeteria. I would go eat with the old people...baked fish, cooked carrots and green beans, mashed potatoes with no gravy, bread (no butter), and water (no soda or juices or caffeinated beverages). This dietary change helped a little.

It wasn't, however, until I rid myself of my inner stress that my stomach pains went away. My mental and emotional turmoil was making my gut roil and boil (I am not known for good poetry). Psychological stress was cured—this was a miracle for me. That second spell of IBS was cured when I quit college; the first spell of IBS was healed when I returned to my faith. Since those early days where IBS pain was a barometer of my stress, I have learned to listen to the brain in my gut...my gut feelings...in the pit

> **Tidbit:**
> I am trained and board-certified as a Family Medicine physician. In days past, we would have been called GPs (general practitioners). I have noticed over my years of training and experience that many GPs acknowledge the role of stress in causing and/or being related to many health maladies, such as spastic colon IBS, stomach ulcers, migraine and tension headaches, high blood pressure...just to name a few. When the gut brain is not happy, the human is not happy or healthy.

Holy and Wholistic Health!

> ### Psycho-somatic? Psycho-spirito-somatic?
> When stress is a primary or secondary cause of physical symptoms, some use the term psychosomatic—meaning the psychological (nephesh soul) thoughts and feelings are producing physical symptoms in the body (soma, somatic). If the soul (brain-mind-heart-feelings) can induce physical feelings, either negative or positive, wouldn't it stand to reason any abnormalities or disturbances in a person's spirit (spirit-soul or soul-spirit) could also generate symptoms in the body?

of my stomach...and make changes accordingly. The lesson for me was if my gut is talking to me, the Lord is communicating with me. This usually involves making a change and finding a way to release the stress that has built up in my life. It has been a good barometer for me so far.

In an earlier section, I mentioned many believe that the conscience of a person is found in the person's spirit. Conscience is a NT Greek word (not found in the OT Hebrew). One definition I found on an internet search defined conscience as "an inner feeling or voice viewed as acting as a guide to the rightness or wrongness of one's behavior." An inner voice or feeling that helps determine right and wrong...I believe this is a fair and accurate definition of a person's conscience. Unlike conscious (consciousness), which is a similar term about being awake and aware, the term conscience has at its core a concept of right and wrong.

> ### Christian Pearl:
> For a Christian, it is so, so, so important to continually let the inner conscience be educated, formed, and developed by constant interactions with God's Word and God's Spirit. A healthy, robust, vibrant, non-violated conscience can be a source of good health and well-being.

The Christian Bible has a lot to say about the conscience of a person. The conscience is a supremely important faculty and determinant of inner health and peace...and potentially psycho-spirito-somatic bodily symptoms. The Bible mentions a good conscience...a pure conscience... not violating the conscience...and much more. If a person's conscience is violated—whether their conscience has been formed from a healthy

Stomach and Intestines

spiritual foundation or not—it can potentially cause many negative soul and body symptoms and conditions.

Bowels and the Inner Man

Let's dive a little deeper (sorry about that) and talk about bowels. Bowels. What a word. I had to look this one up. In the OT, bowels are usually translated from the Hebrew word *me'ah*; in the NT, it is often derived from the Greek word *splagchnon*.

> **Tidbit:**
>
> In medical training, the Latin word *splanchnic* is defined as relating to the internal organs (viscera), especially the abdomen. In this case, the Latin term *splanchnic* is derived originally from Greek.
>
> **Related Tidbit:**
>
> In modern English, the term *visceral* is often used when referring to experiencing something at the deepest level of the gut...at the deepest level of one's being. For instance, it might be said, "_____ (fill in the blank with something extremely unpleasant) produced a visceral response in him..."

Me'ah and *splagchnon* in the Scriptures are mostly used when referring to internal organs, intestines, belly, digestion; in essence, the inward parts. In Scripture, interestingly, the bowels are regarded as the seat of the more violent passions such as love and anger and hate and distress, as well as the deeper positive emotions such as tender affections, kindness, and compassion. It is no wonder that some translations will replace the word *bowels* with *heart*. I guess the authors of the Scriptures (ultimately God) knew about the correlation between the brain in the gut and feelings.

> **Gross Tidbit:**
>
> I suspect that most people have certain triggers that produce a deeply negative visceral response in them, even to the point of being nauseating. I have those triggers. Most of my nauseating visceral triggers have to do with unpleasant smells.

Moved With Compassion...in the Bowels

In the NT era, the Greeks regarded the bowels (*splachna*) as the place where strong and powerful emotions originated. In the OT era, the Hebrews regarded *me'ah* (bowels) as the place where tender mercies and feelings of affection, compassion, sympathy, and pity originated. The Greek word *splanchnizomai* is defined by Strong's Concordance as "to be moved with deep compassion or pity...it is the direct motive for at least 5 of Jesus' miracles." (This paragraph is from *The Spirit-Filled Life Bible*, NKJV, "Word Wealth," p. 1317.) Jesus was often moved with compassion in His bowels to do the good things He did.

> **Bowel Miracle:**
>
> Matthew 14:14 says, *"And when Jesus went out He saw a great multitude; and He was moved with compassion for them, and healed their sick."*
>
> **Another Gut Miracle:**
>
> *"Then Jesus, moved with compassion, stretched out His hand and touched him, and said to him, 'I am willing; be cleansed.' As soon as He had spoken, immediately the leprosy left him, and he was cleansed"* (Mark 1:41-42).

Imagine that...Jesus, the Son of God (and the son of man)...had emotions. At times He allowed His sanctified emotions to lead Him in doing supernatural things. We are to be like Him. If we will submit our emotions to Him, He might also at times lead us by deep, inner emotions. Some of the greatest miracles I have personally witnessed were the result of being deeply moved with compassion. I'm tearing up even now as I write this.

The Touchy-Feely Gut Brain

When referring to the brain in the gut, more often the implication is not that the gut is thinking (per se), as brain neurons think. More often, the implication is that the extensive nerve system of the gut has more of a *feeling* ability, sensing discomfort and dysfunction and pain. The gut is a feeler.

Stomach and Intestines

In contrast to the gut, thinking in the central nervous system is attributed to the brain. It is commonly taught that the brain neurons do not have the ability to feel sensations—no pain receptors or sensory receptors. In the nervous system, which includes the brain, feeling is often attributed to the peripheral nerves that leave the brain and spine and traverse through the body, detecting sensations, pain, hot, cold, itching, burning...any and all sensations.

> ### Related Feeler Tidbit:
> As previously mentioned in another section, the human heart contains as many as 40,000 neurons. Some have called the heart the third brain...the brain in the heart.

Fun Scriptural Examples:

Here are a few fun references of bowel feelings and visceral emotions from the King James Bible. In Philemon 1:20, Paul says, *"...refresh my bowels in the Lord"* (that's one of my favorites). In Colossians 3:12 Paul says, *"Put on... bowels of mercies..."*; in Philippians 1:8, he says, *"...how greatly I long after you all in the bowels of Jesus Christ."* Genesis 43:40 says of Joseph, *"...his bowels did yearn upon his brother"*; Job says, *"My bowels boiled, and rested not..."* (v.30:27; perhaps he had IBS...probably something far worse); Jeremiah says, *"My bowels, my bowels! I am pained at my very heart..."* (v.4:19) and *"my bowels are troubled, my liver is poured upon the earth..."* (Lamentations 2:11). There are many more. You get the idea.

Personal Private Tidbit:

I have been a Christian believer for many years. As a believer, there are many ways to encounter God, such as Bible study and prayer, singing and worship, being thankful, and meeting with other believers. At times when I encounter God's presence, I simultaneously notice physical sensations. During some of the strongest God encounters that produced physical sensations in my body, I experienced sensations primarily in my belly...almost like experiencing electricity...somewhat pleasant and somewhat painful at the same time.

Liver and Kidneys

"The Inner Man?"

I partially quoted Lamentations 2:11 (KJV) in the previous section. Here is a longer quote from that verse: *"Mine eyes do fail with tears, my bowels are troubled, my liver is poured out on the earth..."*

This verse says that his liver was poured upon the earth. In this case, his liver was not poured out; it remained just fine in his body. Jeremiah, the writer of Lamentations, was lamenting with deep sorrow, and this

> ### Tidbit:
> As mentioned briefly already, the anatomical term viscera refer to the internal organs in the main cavities of the body, especially those in the abdomen, including the liver, kidneys, and intestines...and pancreas and spleen...and others.
>
> ### Liver Tidbits:
> The liver is one of the main bodily pathways to remove unwanted toxins and excretor of unwanted metabolic waste into the gut. To name a few other functions of the liver: It produces bile (which aids in digestion), is a producer of certain proteins and cholesterol, is an enzyme activator, and it is a storage facility of fat and glycogen and some vitamins and minerals. The liver is a utility player (to use a sports analogy). The liver is one of those parts that is wildly important but doesn't get a lot of credit.

was how he expressed his sorrow. Some of the non-GI organs that aid in digestion—such as the liver—biblically are often interchanged with the actual digestive organs when referring to the inner parts or inner man or the bowels, especially when relating to deep-seated emotions.

Reins and *kilya* are OT Hebrew words often translated as kidneys. They are often used in describing deep-seated emotions or thoughts, sometimes used interchangeably with the English concepts of mind or heart. Psalm 16:7 says, *"...my reins (kidneys) also instruct me in the night seasons"* (KJV). Psalm 26:2 says, *"Examine me, O Lord...try my mind and my heart..."* In this verse, mind is *kilya* (kidneys) and is considered a place of (what we moderns would classify as) producing inner thought.

The gut and associated internal digestive-related organs are considered as some of the more "undesirables" of the body, necessary gross parts and

Tidbit:
A healthcare slang word for kidney is bean (kidneys would be the plural beans), referring to the overall shape of a kidney resembling a bean. Perhaps that is how the kidney bean got its name?

More Kidney Tidbits:
When I think of kidney function, I think of the obvious removal of unwanted toxins and metabolic wastes from the body by a filtering mechanism—urine. The kidneys also have many other important physiological functions, including maintaining fluid and electrolyte and pH balance, helping regulate blood pressure, and production of certain hormones.

OT Echoes:
When the priests were preparing an animal for a ceremonial sacrifice before the Lord in the OT, they were required to remove the blood and the fat and the kidneys and large lobe of the liver. The liver and kidneys, which in OT thought was considered the seat of the innermost man (often used interchangeably with heart and mind), were also considered sacred and holy to the Lord.

Liver and Kidneys

not to be publicly focused on much for the sake of propriety. However, the gut has many super-important qualities, both physically and biblically...a visceral brain...emotions, passions, thoughts...a germ factory...along with the viaduct of nutrition. When the bowels and internal organs are functioning properly, it leads to good health and a good flow of energy and strength and vitality absent of disease and dysfunction, producing maximum well-being now and (hopefully) for many years to come.

Now turning to that super-fun and super-interesting master...the brain.

BRAINS

Brains

"The Thoughts of Life"

This section on the brains and the thoughts and the mind is gonna be fun! Before we delve into this subject, a few thoughts (haha) that I have: Can I do my own brain surgery? Or, if not, can I at least do my own brain treatments?

In the last section on the bread—the gut—I mentioned the concept of the gut being the second brain of the body. If there is a second, there must be a first...a gold standard...an original that all others are compared to. In this case, the original would be the place where an estimated 86-100 billion neurons reside—the brain. Compare this to an estimated 500 million neurons in the gut. The brain wins.

> **Associated Tidbit Repeated:**
> As mentioned previously, the human heart might have as many as 40,000 neurons. Some have called the heart the third brain...the brain in the heart.

> **Tidbit:**
> Most Google searches on higher education report that psychology is in the top ten majors chosen in college; some sources list it in the top five. I thoroughly enjoyed my undergraduate course in psychology...and my medical school rotation in psychiatry.

The brain—with the accompanying mind—has always been a source of fascination for me. The brain is fascinating for almost all who study it. The study of the brain and mind looks at so many realities... behavior, memory, thoughts,

> **A Muse:**
> I've often wondered if so many students are drawn to psychology not only because it's fascinating but because they are trying to understand how the mind works...in particular how (and maybe why) their own mind works. They may be trying to figure themselves out. I must say, my psychiatry rotation was very eye-opening for me, helping to shed light on some of my past. Scary. Knowledge is not always pleasant.

sleep, dementia...so many important concepts flow from the brain and the mind.

The Thoughts of Life

Now to set the ground rules for this discussion. The human brain is the physical substance...the structure that resembles a very enlarged walnut and is the consistency of firm jelly. It weighs about three pounds, is made up of about 75% water, roughly the size of two clenched fists put together,

> **Malodorous Tidbit:**
> My nose still evokes visceral flashbacks to dissecting a human cadaver in med school...the dominating and overwhelming smell of formaldehyde that the bodies are preserved in. Formaldehyde is an organic solvent and a preservative. There are many organic solvents, and some of the other organic solvents have rather pleasant smells, such as ether and acetone (and for some people gasoline). Formaldehyde is not one of them; not for my nose anyway.
>
> **Organic Solvent Tidbit:**
> As I mentioned earlier in the book, I did organic chemistry research in college. My organic chem professor seemed to hate me but asked me to do summer research with him because his tradition was to ask the person who had the highest score in organic chem to be his summer research assistant. I would spend three afternoon hours in a hot, non-air-conditioned laboratory...think mad scientist images from movies...washing beakers and flasks and other lab paraphernalia with soap and hot water and then chemically

> (Cont): purifying them with acetone and ether so they were usable for experiments. I would inhale the somewhat pleasant volatile solvents acetone and ether all afternoon and then go home with a headache. My wife would tell me she could smell acetone and ether on my breath during most of the evening as I would slowly exhale these floral solvents.

and is something that health students can remove from a (hopefully) dead person and dissect and examine thoroughly.

As the brain is the physical organ, the mind is the more esoteric, invisible part of the mind-brain combination. Somehow, the mind-brain generates thoughts. And the thoughts...well, thoughts are...hard to explain.

Can I Do My Own Brain Surgery?
(Or At Least My Own Brain Treatments?)

Neuroplasticity. There, I said it. One of the hottest current topics in brain science. Neuroplasticity is, in essence, the ability of the brain cells, the neurons, to form new connections between other brain cells—and for the brain to be able to destroy and unhitch and uncouple and re-organize old brain connections that no longer seem useful. As brain-to-brain cell connections appear to be the pathway on which thoughts travel, the ability to continually re-structure brain pathways is one of the more powerful tools the brain has. Think (pun) of the obvious benefits of neuroplasticity after suffering brain damage with a stroke or head injury or in someone experiencing a debilitating neurological disease such as Parkinson's or dementia.

Physical brain specialists (neurologists, neurosurgeons, neuroscientists, and others) and the mind-thought-emotion specialists (psychologists, psychiatrists, therapists, counselors, etc.) all do a wonderful job with the current knowledge available in mind-brain science. There are so many individuals, often personal family and friends, affected by brain afflictions—such as stroke, dementia, Alzheimer's, tumors, Parkinson's, ALS, all forms of mental health, and many other brain problems. Thank you, mind-brain specialists, for all that you do!

Holy and Wholistic Health!

"For as he thinks in his heart, so is he."

The verse above, Proverbs 23:7, is one of my favorite Bible verses. As has been previously discussed, the OT Hebrew often uses interchangeable words and concepts when referring to the heart and the mind and thoughts. The far-reaching ramifications of this verse—as a person thinks, so they are—implies that our thoughts determine our behavior, our identity, the very essence of who we are. And with neuroplasticity, our thoughts change the structure, patterns, and circuits of our brains.

> **Tidbit:**
> Dr. Caroline Leaf is a cognitive neuroscientist who has written extensively on how our thoughts change our brains. I recommend her books for those wanting to dive deeper into her brain-changing research.

My goal—and hopefully yours—is to keep intentionally aligning my thoughts with good things...peace...joy...happiness...the Word of God... choosing positive, healthy thoughts that will change my brain...essentially, doing my own brain surgery daily (surgery being used here loosely as something that alters tissue structure)...more appropriately worded, essentially doing my own brain treatments that bring structural brain change on a daily basis! I intentionally endeavor to think positive, healthy thoughts and reject and dismiss negative thoughts that are toxic to health.

> **Correlated Verse:**
> "...be transformed by the renewing of your mind..." Romans 12:2. Another version quotes this as "...let God transform you into a new person by changing the way you think." (NLT) Obviously, this verse speaks to changing one's behavior; I believe it also applies to brain transformation.
>
> **Another Verse Paraphrased:**
> "Think on these things...whatever is true, noble, just, pure, lovely...of good report...virtuous and praiseworthy things...meditate on these things." (Philippians 4:8).

I want to give neuroplasticity a chance to work in my favor for healthy brain changes...daily. Every day.

Who knew that something as simple and easy as thinking the thoughts of God would allow me to do my own daily brain treatments?

Does Exercise Help?

I recently came across a TED Talk by Wendy Suzuki, a professor of neuroscience and psychology, that discussed an inexpensive and relatively easy way to promote a healthy brain and mind—exercise. From her research, she asserts that regular exercise improves all things brain and mind, including but not limited to memory, alertness, mood, and attention—by not only physiologically improving the brain but also by anatomically and chemically changing the brain. Based on all that I have read and experienced, I believe she is correct. Exercise can be another form of doing self-brain therapy that alters brain structure and function for the better. Her TED Talk can be found at the TED Talk website under "The brain-changing benefits of exercise" by Wendy Suzuki.

Personal Tidbit:

I discovered many years ago that when I have a reading assignment...information or material I need to process and think through...that I tend to be more successful in my processing if I am walking while reading. My brain seems to be more alive, creative, and optimistic if I am moving my whole body while reading...getting my blood flowing...constantly changing the background scenery...getting fresh air when outside.

Learning to Walk Before You Run Tidbit:

I enjoyed walk-reading so much that I experimented with the next level—I tried jogging and reading. I liked it even better! Over the last 18 years of jog-walk reading, I have only fallen three times that I remember (insert crazy-face emoji with tongue hanging out here). No serious injuries. I finally learned to enjoy and look forward to reading again after many years of stationary, stale reading.

Sleep

"Life's Regular Time-Out"

"When you lie down, your sleep will be sweet."
Proverbs 3:24 (AMP)

I always thought (pun) if I had gone into research, I probably would have studied sleep as one of my topics. I find it incredible that humans need regular episodes of becoming essentially unconscious to be healthy...and feel good...and not be grumpy...and have energy. It's as if humans must undergo regular mini-hibernation spells of dormancy. Not experiencing these regular times of dormancy is not optional for good health and a sound mind.

In this discussion, I will not focus on sleep disorders; thank goodness we have very talented and well-trained sleep specialists to diagnose and treat sleep problems. Thank you, sleep specialists, for all that you do!

Sweet Sleep

Studying what actually happens when a person sleeps—the stages of sleep—is something I regularly cycle back around to in my thoughts and readings. The transitional first stage of sleep is sort of like being awake and asleep simultaneously. Then you drop into stage two with its electrical spindles; the spindles are almost like a lighthouse or a transmitter that sends regular pulses throughout the brain. In stages three and four, a person goes on into the deeper, healing stages of sleep, where everything seems to shut down, offline if you will—and then into the crazy, zany world of REM dreaming where the brain is super-active, and the body remains (hopefully) paralyzed. The sleeper will then cycle back and forth throughout the night in and out of these different sleep phases before waking up feeling, hopefully, refreshed, re-charged, and ready to go. Sleep stages are mysterious and fun to ponder.

Taking Out the Brain Trash

Sleep science continues to research and deep dive into not only what is happening during sleep but why we require sleep. New discoveries surface regularly.

A more recent and eye-opening discovery theorizes that during the deeper levels of sleep, the brain tissue relatively shrinks, allowing the fluid which bathes the brain (the cerebrospinal fluid) to flow more freely through the brain structures and then back out into the body's general circulation, thus allowing the breakdown products of brain activity...cellular debris...toxins...trash, if you will...to be removed.

Healthy sleep cleanses the brain and keeps unwanted substances from building up and causing dysfunction, which seems to have tremendous implications for dementia disorders. Said another way, according to this theory, healthy sleep detoxes the brain.

A Good Night's Sleep Recharges the Batteries

> **Personal Friend Tidbit:**
> My long-time friend Keven likes to say to me as I am dropping him off at his home in the evening, "I hope you have a good sleep."

The deeper stages of sleep are believed to be a central focus of when the brain—and the rest (pun) of the body—goes through a phase of cleansing, as well as healing, restoring, and re-charging. The simultaneous cleansing out the brain trash along with healthy restoration (such as releasing

Sleep

> **Tidbit:**
> *Sleep pressure* refers to the feeling of being sleepy and increases as the day goes on. It is believed that sleep pressure results from the accumulation of adenosine, a break-down chemical of cellular metabolism, in the brain. Adenosine has sleep-inducing effects. Sleep helps remove the adenosine build-up, allowing one to feel refreshed and "good to go" after a good night's sleep or a power nap.

health-promoting hormones) is designed to produce growth and energy. The body's physiology is designed, if working properly, so a person wakes up healthier and with new reserves of energy. More vigor. More vitality. Healthier and stronger.

In my previous discussions, the soul of man is considered both the invisible (mind, emotions, and thoughts) and the visible (brain and body). Healthy sleep restores and re-invigorates both mind and body! The spirit-soul force of a human is designed to be replenished with a good sleep...or even a good nap.

> **A Favorite Verse:**
> *"The Lord...He makes me to lie down... He restores my soul"* (Psalm 23:1-3).
>
> **Another Fav Verse:**
> *"When you lie down, your sleep will be sweet..."* (Proverbs 3:24 AMP). (In this particular passage, sweet sleep is the result of the one who finds wisdom and discretion and applies said wisdom in their life.)

Deep sleep seems to induce a hibernation-like effect. Unconscious deep sleep has many similarities to being in a coma, even being close to death—or even an anesthesia-like effect, such as when God caused a deep sleep to fall upon Adam so he could do surgery and remove a rib (Gen 2:21). It blows my mind (a punn-ish cliché) that we must regularly become comatose-like in order to maintain good health. Incidentally, the Scriptures are notorious for using the word sleep when referring to death.

> **Fun Tidbit:**
>
> The Bible records many instances of the word *sleep* being used to refer to death, more than I want to mention. A fun story connects the concepts of sleep and death...Paul was preaching a marathon sermon, and a young boy fell asleep...and then fell out of a high window and died (not a fun story yet). As if seemingly an almost routine occurrence, Paul went down and prayed for the boy, and he came back to life. Ho hum, another person raised from the dead.

A Troubled Mind, A Troubled Heart

I have mentioned earlier that family doctors, myself included, are notorious for acknowledging the mind-body connection and how it affects health and well-being. During sleep, human bodies need to heal and restore...but the inner man, the soul, the mind, and inner heart need to also find rest. For the inner man, the soul, healing rest does not have to be while asleep. An awake and conscious person can be experiencing rest for the heart and mind; peace would be another good synonym for rest. Shalom is another.

> **Interesting Tidbit:**
>
> The inner man—mind, heart, soul, spirit—has already been discussed at length. An interesting concept to me is that the innermost man, whatever that is (spirit? soul?) can be active while the physical body is sleeping, as evidenced in the verse, *"I sleep, but my heart is awake..."* (Song of Solomon 5:2).

One roadblock to getting good, healthy sleep is stress. Stress. That word is a power-packed word. Stress can be positive—good and healthy, like exercising or fasting. Or stress can be negative—unhealthy and debilitating. Now diving a little deeper into how stress can affect sleep...

Sleep

> **Pearl:**
> In the many stages of my sleep...especially when I'm in a lighter stage of sleep...I have sorted out problems and found solutions to conundrums that were not obvious while I was awake. As a Christian believer, I understand my inner man, in these sleep stages, is interacting with me—my soul and spirit...my "self"—and also with the Spirit of God. Heaven and earth are coming together!

Where Did My Sleep Go?

Stress that leads to worry, fear, or anxiety can cause a person's sleep to flee, creating insomnia. Insomnia can be a lack of sleep or prolonged difficulty falling asleep...no sleep or tossing and turning in non-restorative sleep. Not good either way for living in good health.

When I'm not sleeping due to inner turmoil—whatever the cause—I will do whatever is necessary to get my sleep restored...physical remedies... habit adjustments...soul-heart changes...repentance...whatever. At my age, there's too much on the line; lack of sleep has an association with increased risks of diabetes, heart disease, and dementia (just to name a few). I've got to get my zzz's.

> **Lion King Insomnia:**
> Apparently, King Darius of Persia's conscience was bothering him when he knowingly had innocent Daniel thrown to the lions. Daniel 6:18 records that *"...the King went to his palace, and spent the night fasting... (and) his sleep went from him."* God intervened for Daniel when a pagan, yet God-fearing, king succumbed to his own pride and threw an innocent man to the ferocious meat-lovers. Could the fact the same pagan king fasted for Daniel have helped bring about God's divine intervention for Daniel?

Memory

"The Replay of Life"

But I Can't Remember...

Along with lack of sleep or poor-quality sleep being associated with increased risks of diabetes and heart disease, current research seems to confirm a strong association with healthy sleep and strong memory; said in reverse...there is a correlation between poor sleep and poor memory, apparently being a key component of the multifactorial dementia processes.

The Memory-Sleep Connection

I love to read current scientific findings on sleep and how it affects memory. A current theory seems to go as follows: We are continuously interacting with the world while awake, receiving all manner of sensory, physical, intellectual, and social input...all incoming data is temporarily stored in short-term memory centers whether we were consciously aware of the input or not. When we fall asleep, the early phases of sleep, probably stage 2, start to unload the new input data into other areas of the brain that are capable of storage into longer-term memory...and then—wham, pow, voila—when we start to dream in REM sleep, our brains somehow begin to consolidate all of the new input from the day into our already established functioning brain. Is the new inputted memory data stored and placed in our brain randomly? Smartly? By association? Is this why

> **Tidbit:**
> Some studies seem to indicate that if a student is studying new information—as in getting ready to take a test—and then takes a nap, the information is better retained.

dreams often have elements of today's experiences intertwined with old experiences, forming a surreal dream experience?

And then, if dream consolidation is successful because of healthy sleep, we have new memories recorded in long-term brain storage. There, you have it. Dr. Clark's (paraphrased) understanding of memory in a nutshell. Fascinating! (Note: What is fas-

Interesting:

Stage 2 of sleep is known for sleep spindles. I have heard sleep spindles explained by different sleep experts with not all experts arriving at the same conclusions. Be that as it may, here is what seems to be happening with sleep spindles: Neuro-electrical spikes shoot through the brain in a mostly patterned way...but for what purpose(s)? My simple mind (pun intended) sees these as electrical impulses of neuronal energy almost like a beacon sends out rays of light in all directions, pulsing regularly. But again, for what purpose(s)? Whatever sleep spindles are accomplishing, stage 2 has been described as the go-between phase all night long between deep restorative sleep (stages 3 and 4) and REM dream sleep. For instance, a phase of deep sleep...followed by a phase of stage 2 sleep spindles...followed by a phase of REM dreaming...followed by a phase of stage 2 sleep spindles...and so on. Of all the many purposes of sleep spindles, some sort of consolidation and preparation and adjustments seem to be taking place. My suspicion is sleep spindles affect memory consolidation at some important level.

Personal:

When falling asleep, I love being aware of the oncoming sleep stages... knowing I will most likely go through a semi-lucid stage 1, in which I might be somewhat consciously aware...followed by the riveting pulses of stage 2 sleep spindles, that are apparently doing something really good for my brain and mind...

Memory

cinating is not my explanation but the memory concepts themselves and especially how sleep plays a strong role in memory creation.)

Anything that interferes with healthy sleep—stress, fatigue, pain, illness, inner turmoil, physical deformities, sleep apnea, medications (even sleep medications that induce sleep but do not guarantee that all sleep stages will be healthy and adequate)—can disrupt the "memory-zation" process (my term, as if that's not obvious). Disrupted memory consolidation over time is instrumental in dementia processes such as Alzheimer's.

Healthy Interventions:
Along with healthy sleep contributing to preventing dementia and Alzheimer's, other interventions have been shown to be beneficial to prevent dementia and Alzheimer's, such as regular aerobic exercise, eating a heart healthy diet, and learning new things. Lisa Genova, a neuroscientist and author, has explained this in greater detail in her TED Talk.[1]

Disrupted sleep might help explain why some individuals suffer from poor memory, such as my wonderful mother who was able to remember things in great detail that happened many years ago but couldn't remember what happened five minutes ago. Her short-term memory consolidation machinery was not functioning properly. Another observation about my mom: I have also noticed she could remember and sing songs from her past with great precision but then have difficulty with recent details and simple current conversation.

Divine Pearl:
Man's spirit connection with God's Spirit can be helpful in memory recall. John 14:26 says it this way: *"But the Helper, the Holy Spirit...He will teach you all things, and bring to your remembrance all things I said to you."* In my own life, I have found that God's Spirit will not only teach me but help me with the power of recall by accessing brain areas where information has already been stored.

---

[1] Lisa Genova's TED Talk, "What you can do to prevent Alzheimer's": https://podcasts.google.com/feed/aHR0cHM6Ly9mZWVkcyIuZmVlZGJ1cm5lci5jb20vdGVkdGFsa3NfYXVkaW8/episode/ZW4uYXVkaW8udGFsay50ZWQuY29tOjI3NzE=?ep=14

Holy and Wholistic Health!

> **Personal Tidbit:**
>
> Knowing this truth helped me get through pre-med and med school (and still helps me today). When I would take a (stressful) test...knowing that a failing F grade on a med school test would get me kicked out of school, and knowing that stress and worry would short-circuit my power or recall...I would sit and pray and ask for divine recall help as the test papers were being handed out. It seemed to work. And I enjoyed taking tests more!
>
> ....
>
> **Another Personal Tidbit:**
>
> My wonderful mother, who has since passed away, was diagnosed with Alzheimer's dementia. When I talked to her, she was usually happy and smiling. What she said sometimes made sense, and she loved to sing with me, especially Jesus songs. Her physical brain was certainly dysfunctional. Her mind-soul was in and out...coming and going. Her spirit? Her spirit seemed to be intact. Seemed to be just fine!

Do not let anything interfere with healthy sleep. The potential cost to one's health and brain and memory is too high. Think the thoughts of God. Do your own brain surgery treatments. Live a long and happy life with good energy and vitality with a sound mind and body.

Now let's turn and see how the body's supporting structures can lead to good health, energy, and vitality.

Memory

Another Comment:

For whatever it's worth, Mom did have trouble sleeping for many years. As long as I can remember, she took medicine to help her sleep. Sleep medication may put someone into some form of sleep but does not guarantee healthy, restorative sleep.

And Also:

Mom's memory brain problem is a mystery. I heard Pastor Paul Manwaring say, in regard to the mystery side of Jesus and God, the following tenants which have helped me: God is good; He is here; Jesus won ultimate victory; nothing is impossible; every individual is significant; and there is mystery. Well said.

Final Note:

Mom passed away after her long struggle with memory problems. I had the privilege of being with her as her spirit-soul left her dysfunctional body. Her breathing stopped (spirit, lungs, air)…then her eyelids closed…then her heart stopped beating. She is now in the arms of Jesus!

BONES

In this section, I would like to delve into the supporting structure of the human body—the bones, muscles, tendons, ligaments—and see how they can support (pun) good health, energy, and vitality. I am referring to all these supporting structures under the umbrella term "Bones."

The concept of calling the outer supporting framework structure bones is not unique or new with me. I heard a well-known HGTV personality say that a particular house had good bones but just needed some TLC renovation. Similar phrases could be used in referring to the outer shell framework of a car.

An obvious statement I will make here: Poor health, a poor quality of life, can certainly come from the malfunctioning of the internal engine parts of a human such as the brain, heart, lungs, and digestion. Other people can have healthy "internal engine systems" running and yet have a poor quality of life due to a deteriorating outer framework.

A clunky analogy of this...My son's first car was a 30-year-old small Toyota truck and legitimately had only 30,000 miles on it. The engine purred like a kitten, and it ran great! The problem? The plastics and rubber supporting parts kept falling apart...door handles would break...door locks would malfunction...the outer framework materials could not stand the wear-and-tear test of time.

Bones

"The Framework of Life"

Just as a well-built house must have a solid framework of concrete, wood, and/or steel (and other materials), the human body must have an underlying solid framework on which to build the rest of the structure. The basic underlying solid structures of the body are the bones.

Human bone cells (osteocytes) include calcium in their make-up. Bones—especially the long bones of the arms and legs and also the spinal column—give other supporting structures a lattice work in which the body can support itself and take shape.

> **Fact:**
>
> The outer perimeter of a bone is where the firm, hardness of the bone is located. The inner part, the marrow, is more spongy and hollow and filled with a fat-filled blob of goodness (more on that later).

If bones are "not right" and causing dysfunction, they can be problematic in many different ways. Obviously, bones can be broken, fractured, cracked, and cause pain and a weak or dysfunctional point of support.

> **Trouble:**
>
> Osteoporosis (thinning bones of aging), Paget's disease of the bone, osteogenesis imperfecta, Ricketts, osteonecrosis, osteoarthritis, bone infections, and bone tumors are just some of the many bone abnormalities that can cause structural problems.

Holy and Wholistic Health!

Positive Verses:

A few scriptural examples of how the bones can be positively impacted for good health: *"it (a right relationship with God)... will be health to your flesh (literally your navel), and strength to your bones"* (Proverbs 3:8). *"And a good report makes the bones healthy (literally fat)"* (Proverbs 15:30). *"Pleasant words are like a honeycomb, sweetness to the soul and health to the bones"* (Proverbs 16:24).

Or, bones can be diseased or improperly formed, none of which is healthy.

The OT Hebrew word for bone is `etsem. Many OT Bible verses speak of inner heart turmoil negatively affecting one's `etsem, one's bones. A few examples include how a wrong relationship with God can harm bones and other organs: *"When I kept silent, my bones grew old through my groaning all the day long"* (Psalm 32:3). *"...all my bones are out of joint; my heart is like wax; it has melted within me"* (Psalm 22:14). *"...grief... sighing...my strength fails...my bones waste away..."* (Psalm 31:10). *"There is no soundness in my flesh...nor any health in my bones..."* (Psalm 38:3). *"My bones are burned like a hearth...because of...my groaning my bones cling to my skin"* (Psalm 102:3,5). *"...envy is rottenness to the bones"* (Proverbs 14:30).

I find it fascinating (I feel like I say that a lot) that the blood cells of life—the white and red blood cells and the platelets—are manufactured in the spongy, hollow-ish spaces inside the hard, outer shell of the bones. It's as if the design (wink) of the bone is such that these most precious life-blood cells are conceived, incubated, and cocooned in one of the safest places of the body. Also fascinating is that these cells are surrounded by fat cells, unhealthy in excess yet a healthy insulation for the cells of life. Brilliant!

Proverbs 3:8 promises strength in the bones. While writing this paragraph, my wife and I are currently recuperating from Covid. We have both had very mild cases and are doing really well. Praying for healing for my wife and myself, I usually say the prayer that I have offered to many who have had Covid over the last two years: "Lord, breathe Your breath in their lungs and put Your strength in their bones...Your energy in their bones overcoming all fatigue!"

Posture

"Upright Living"

"This only I have found: God created mankind upright..."
Ecclesiastes 7:29 (NIV)

I, like many people, have been through phases in my life where I have experienced low back pain. Often, the cause is either I have gained weight or overworked my back muscles, causing a muscular strain. An old-school term for low back pain is lumbago.

It was during one of my lumbago spells caused by over-straining my low back muscles working at a lumberyard that I decided to pursue a career to become a physician. That is another story for another time. The Lord has led me through many important life-direction decisions, sometimes using my physical symptoms in helping to clarify the direction.

> ### Tidbit:
> Lumbago is a Latin-derived word for low back pain. Back pain is historically one of the top ten reasons why people visit a doctor.
>
> ### Adjustment Tidbit:
> I did an elective rotation while in my Family Medicine Residency with a friend who was a chiropractor. I learned a great deal by observing how he would physically manipulate back muscles and provide relief for those with back pain.

As I have aged, hopefully gracefully, I have found that one of the tools in my tool belt to combat low back strains is to improve my slouching

Holy and Wholistic Health!

> **Psalm 25 Pearl:**
> *"Good and upright is the Lord"* (Psalm 25:8).
>
> **Psalm 26 Also:**
> In Psalm 26, David says, *"...I have walked in my integrity...but as for me, I will walk in my integrity..."* (verses 1 and 11). Integrity correlates to soundness and wholeness and is intimately connected to uprightness of heart and soul.

posture. I had heard improved posture could help with back pain, and I bought a $10 VHS tape called "Pilates for Dummies" and, once having viewed the instructor demonstrating the non-ball floor exercises, scoffed at how easy this was going to be. WRONG! Those exercises proverbially kicked my backside.

Long story shorter...some of the exercises were actually making my back hurt. So, I systematically eliminated exercises that seemed to be hurting my back...from around 28 exercises down to 3 or 4. I began to notice that my "modified Pilates" exercises actually made my back feel better, and they helped my belly not pooch out as much and helped me straighten my back. Better posture!

> **More Psalm 25:**
> *"Let integrity and uprightness preserve me"* (Psalm 25:21).

I learned about other stretches and exercises for better posture and began to implement them. I heard many anecdotal stories that even purported better overall health from better posture. Some reports promised that a person would look leaner when they stood up straight. I think they might be onto something. I do feel leaner when I stand up straighter.

One day as I was pondering my Bible readings, I came across Ecclesiastes 7:29 which states, *"God made mankind upright..."* On this particular day, that phrase especially caught my attention. God made man upright. I do not read in the creation story of Genesis of God making any of the other animals upright. Even some of the animals we observe that can stand or walk upright, such as apes and monkeys, possess a natural posture that is

Posture

> **Hebrew Nerding-Out:**
> The Hebrew word *upright* in Ecclesiastes 7:29 is translated as the word *yashar*, which is also used as straight...right...level...correct...proper. It is also used in conjunction with having an uprightness of man's inner heart. Being upright in heart possesses a moral rightness component that is beautiful and healthy...face up, properly inclined toward God (many verses could be cited, especially in the Psalms and Proverbs).

face toward the ground on all four legs. Much could be inferred from this observation. Man was made in God's image.

As man is a soul-spirit designed to become a spirit-soul (see the earlier sections on theology for more details), a few things stick out to me that separates man from the animals, such as (1) man was created upright, (2) God breathed His breath of life into man's lungs (see earlier sections), and (3) God put eternity in man's heart (Ecclesiastes 3:11). In man's soul-spirit, there are other distinctions, but these have significantly impacted my thinking.

Inclination and Attitude

A concept term that is closely related to posture is attitude. One definition of attitude related to posture is "a position of the body." Apparently, the origin of the word *attitude* was a French word denoting the placing or posture of a figure in art. However, a more complete definition of attitude is "a position of the body...proper to or implying an action or mental state."

> **Bible Verse:**
> *"Have this same attitude in yourselves which was in Christ Jesus..."* (Philippians 2:5). The AMP and NASB versions use the actual word attitude. Most of the other versions use *mind* in place of attitude.

This more comprehensive definition of attitude brings out the connection of position with the inner man's mental state. Attitude, as understood in modern vernacular, has to do with the inner man's heart position.

Holy and Wholistic Health!

I am an airplane nerd. I like to watch airplanes fly. Especially the big ones like the Boeing 747 and the Airbus 380. Any of the wide-body airplanes are good for me; the bigger the better. One of my favorite forms of inexpensive recreation at home is to watch live airplanes taking off on YouTube (many YouTube channels have live plane spotting at the bigger airports). I also like to watch and study an airplane app on my phone that tracks all planes in the air, noting their speeds, altitudes, where the flight originated, and the arrival destination. My wife makes fun of me for all this airplane nerding-out.

There is an aviation definition of attitude that has to do with position. Without a lengthy discussion or definition, which I would probably get wrong, the attitude of an airplane has to do with its position in space relative to the earth's horizon (not a complete definition). Terms such as an airplane's pitch, roll, and yaw help define an airplane's position in relation to the earth.

It helps my simple mind to understand the term attitude by another word—inclination. The airplane has an inclination in regard to the earth. My body has an inclination in regard to gravity and space. My heart and inner man have an inclination in regard to everything around it. Using me as an example, the inclination of my heart is the attitude of my heart.

Do I Need an Adjustment?

I don't know about you, but, from time to time, I have needed an adjustment of my attitude. If the inclination of my heart and my mind and my thoughts are not square with reality, not square with what is true, my attitude might start to pitch and roll and yaw. I am not a pilot, but I know that if an airplane's gauges of attitude are not right, especially at night or in poor visibility, a plane could accidentally be flown into the ground or into a mountain.

> **Tidbit:**
> Another obvious reference to posture adjustment is when chiropractors adjust the back and musculo-skeletal system, bringing the body into proper alignment.

> ### Another Bible Concept:
> If my heart attitude is inclined opposite of God and His reality, I might find myself in a biblical state of deception. The heart does have the ability to deceive itself, especially if it is thus inclined. One of my regular prayer phrases is "Lord, keep me back from secret faults, dark spots, blind spots, deceptions, and presumptive sins" (for references to these phrases see Psalm 19:12-13; Luke 11:36; 1 Corinthians 3:18, 6:9, and 15:33; Galatians 6:7; 1 John 1:8; all NKJV).
>
> ### Deception Pearl:
> I have been in deception before; it is not pretty and does not produce good fruit in my life when I am in such an abnormal state of heart and mind inclination. Results of deception may not be evident at first and may, initially, even be very enjoyable and freeing. However, my past bouts of deception, played out over time, became toxic, even in certain situations very destructive and dangerous.

Sometimes, I need to adjust the inclination of my heart attitude. It is always good and helpful and a relief to get re-adjusted properly when I'm off. One biblical word for this is the term repentance. Repentance means to change...to change me...change my heart's attitude...and get my heart's inclination back in line with God and His reality.

I understand that a discussion about attitude could have easily and correctly been placed under the "heart" heading. It would have fit. For whatever reason, I felt it best to put it here under posture.

> ### Health Pearl:
> *"Don't be impressed with your own wisdom. Instead, fear the Lord and turn away from evil. Then you will have healing for your body and strength for your bones"* (Proverbs 3:7 NLT).
>
> ### Longevity Pearl:
> *"She (God's wisdom) offers you long life..."* (Proverbs 3:16 NLT).

Muscles
"The Energy of Life"

Bones obviously play a significant role in posture. To be sure, muscles also play a significant role in posture. When I do Pilates exercises, it is primarily the muscular structures with their associated ligaments and tendons that I am stretching and forming. Muscles, ligaments, and tendons (collectively I will call "muscles") bring pliability in conjunction with the rigidness of bones, completing the overall foundational structure of the outer human body.

Movement and Exercise

I played sandlot sports in my neighborhood growing up and also played school-organized sports until I graduated. Therefore, for fun (community games with friends) and as a requirement (school teams), I exercised. I still get a little queasy when I hear the word wind-sprints. The obvious benefits of exercise, even forced, were good for me and helped keep my weight under control.

Then I graduated. No more forced exercise. You guessed it—upward weight creep.

I began a battle...a quest...a journey...a love-hate relationship with exercise. I would start a routine, highly motivated with strict discipline and success, then my motivation would wane. The exercise would fall by the wayside because of a new job routine. Or a new season in life with dif-

Holy and Wholistic Health!

ferent activities putting new demands on my time. Or the warm summer would turn to cold winter. Or maybe I would just get a little lazy. And the exercise would fall by the wayside. Many years of this.

One day, around my 39th year, I found a routine that I liked. For exercise, I would jog and then walk and then jog and then walk—and repeat indefinitely. I fell in love with this habit and found that I could keep up this pace for long periods of time. And I enjoyed it. I would pray...or read... or listen...often to inspirational material. My jog-walk, which one of my friends calls "the Jon Clark shuffle," became an extension of my morning devotions. Brilliant!

Just Do It!

Move. Exercise. Be active. All forms of muscular exercise produce positive health benefits, be it muscle-building weightlifting or aerobic exercise or job-related occupational activity or recreational hobbies. They're all good

> **Tidbit:**
> When I was struggling over a twenty-year period to find an exercise routine that worked for me, often my discipline would get interrupted during a major life shift that seemed to take priority over exercising. When I discovered my jog-walk shuffle, my commitment to exercise was raised to the level of conviction. In other words, I had to view exercise commitments on a similar discipline level as my spiritual convictions (prayer, worship, Bible study, church attendance)... almost to the point of committing a sin if I did not just do it (exercise). This helped immensely.
>
> **Tidbit Continued:**
> Most weeks, I am able to exercise at least five days per week with my aerobic shuffle and two or three days per week with my modified Pilates. During the summer when the sun comes up earlier and I have more pre-work time, I usually can do the Jon Clark shuffle every day.

> **Divine Echoes:**
> The OT Hebrew word *halak* is defined as to go, to walk, to move. Physical bodily exercise is important for good health. Spirit and soul exercise is also important, as evidenced in the parallel phrases from Psalm 26 where David says, *"I have walked (halak) in my integrity...but as for me, I will walk (halak) in my integrity..."* (verses 1 and 11). See also 1 Timothy 4:7-8 for another reference to the importance of spirit and soul and body exercise.

for health and disease prevention, helping prevent diabetes, high blood pressure, high cholesterol, heart disease, stroke, and many other conditions. Exercise is also good for the overall sense of well-being, which is a part of living in good health. The key to sustaining an exercise routine is to find a routine—a habit that does not damage the body and does not lead to boredom—that can fit into a daily life pattern.

The Knee Bone's Connected to the...

When a bone meets and connects to another bone, a joint is formed. *Harmos* and *arthron* are Greek words for a musculo-skeletal joint. If a compound medical word starts with *artho-*, think joint. Another Latin word for joint is *articulus*. Think *articulus* when one bone articulates with another, forming a joint with another bone. And, most often, the attaching pieces of bones that form a joint are overlaid with cartilage surfaces.

Most boney joints (1) have a soft tissue capsule lining and (2) have ligaments and tendons interacting within the joint. Ligaments are firm bands of durable connective tissue that connect bone to bone, and tendons are similar, maybe a little more pliable, that connect

> **Cartilage Tidbit:**
> Cartilage is a resilient, elastic tissue; a rubber-like yet shiny padding that covers and protects the ends of bones. It is not as rigid as bone and yet is much stiffer and less flexible than muscle. It seems to function as a cap, hopefully allowing the surface of one bone to slide smoothly over the surface of the other bone. Cartilage is also found in other non-joint places such as the nose and the ear.

> ### Fun Verse (Hebrews 4:12):
> *"The word of God is...powerful...sharper than any two-edged sword, piercing even to the division of soul and spirit...of (the) joints (harmos) and marrow (myelos)...is a discerner of the thoughts and intents of the heart."* According to this verse, God's Word can divide the inner man (soul and spirit) and can also divide the outer man (joints and bone marrow).
>
> ### Associated Tidbit:
> The Greek NT word for marrow is *myelos*. In the OT, marrow was often associated with the concepts of being fattened and prosperous. As a reminder, the bone marrow does contain fat cells.

muscle to bone. Mixing rigid strong bones with pliable strong muscles, joints, ligaments, tendons, and elastic cartilage—the basic outer framework of the human body is composed. On and in this outer framework are all the "internals."

Energy—A Big Health Connection

And now for a big health connection. As has already been alluded to, regular exercise helps people feel better overall—more psychologically well, experiencing more overall well-being, health, and more energy! I notice an immediate diminishing of my overall energy on the days I do not exercise. I am not as energetic. I feel sluggish, like I have "energy constipation" (I felt I just had to get that phrase in there). My vitality, vigor, and physical-soul man suffers on the days I do not exercise.

Human energy is a reality, a concept I have been alluding to from many different angles so far. What is energy in a human? We feel it when we have it. In non-biological nature, energy is easily defined by the laws of physics and is a fascinating reality to study and ponder, the essence relating to the ability to do work.

But in biological life systems, and humans in particular, energy as a concept is not as easy to define. Does it relate to the power that is resident in a body builder with large muscles? Does it relate to physiological reserve that is stored up in an athlete that is physically fit? Is it something I can feel when I wake up in the morning and gauge throughout the day? How is it related to food? To sleep? Is it something I am also aware of in my invisible self, my soul and spirit? Are there many other ways human energy could be defined and explained and experienced? The answer is yes to all of these questions.

When referring to living with good health, energy is a king...or at least one of the main components that contribute to good health. A person may be physically healthy in the sense of being free from disease, but, if they lack energy in their body and soul, are they really living healthy? Possessing energy is a big health connection.

Bible Tidbit:

Second Timothy 1:6 says, "...*Stir up the gift of God that is in you...*" I acknowledge now that I will be taking this verse out of context. Guilty. The biblical concept is Timothy had a spiritual gift that had been given to him and was lying mostly dormant; his mentor, Paul, wanted him to stir up that dormant gift again and get it activated.

Related Tidbit:

When I force non-energetic self to exercise in the morning, I am stirring up the gift of energy that is in me!

Another Tidbit:

Human cells have DNA—the genetic code—in the nucleus of the cell. The nucleus is considered the mastermind, the brain if you will, of a cell. However, mitochondria also have their own DNA. No other cellular organelle possesses DNA except mitochondria (along with the nucleus). Not sure of the significance of this, but I can speculate, which is always a good thing to do in science (haha).

Holy and Wholistic Health!

Fun Speculation:

It seems as though DNA...the genetic code...the blueprint for life...is in essence, the very essence of what a human body is. Every person's DNA is what makes them unique. DNA strands are the templates by which proteins are synthesized. Seemingly obvious to me—mitochondrial DNA must likewise be about the process of producing proteins. Perhaps more DNA protein-generating machinery is needed in muscles due to the high energy needs?

Speculation Part 2:

But a human is not just a body. Throughout this writing, I have continually connected the concept of good health with abundance of energy. I have also connected good health with both visible body and invisible soul. Stretch with me (smile) on this—could it be that the soul is, in some way, as dependent upon ATP-generated energy as is the body? DNA bodily essence in the nucleus representing the physical body—and the mitochondria energy producers of the body—could also provide energy for the soul. Body and soul intertwined for good health...both need energy for vitality and vigor.

Muscle Energy—Stir Up the Gift That is in You

When I exercise in the morning, exerting energy, I end up having more overall energy and end up feeling better throughout my day. What gives?

During exercise, muscles that are normally doing the routine work of daily living are recruited to be repetitively used for running, walking, weight-lifting, biking, swimming...whatever the exercise may be. During exercise, the muscle groups that normally are fairly quiet are now called upon to contract and relax...and contract and relax...and contract and relax...over and over and over. This increase in muscle use shifts blood flow to be maximized in the muscle groups being used, along with sending extra blood flow to the heart (providing the blood to the body) and the lungs (providing the oxygen). Increased muscle use during exercise reveals that muscles have energy generators in-house and at the ready.

Muscle Mitochondria

Back to junior high biology class. In human cells, one of the intracellular organelles I remember studying was a goofy looking little structure, often portrayed to have a bean-like shape—the mitochondrion (plural is mitochondria). I looked up the derivative roots of mitochondria and nothing spectacular stuck out to me.

But here's the thing: If you had biology class and listened well, you'll remember mitochondria are the powerhouses of the cell. Within the cells' mitochondria are where energy is produced. And, for those that studied biochemistry or physiology—or just Googled it or are just really smart—you'll remember that the mitochondria produce biological energy in the form of a molecule called ATP. Muscle cells have higher numbers of mitochondria than other cells, making them capable of producing greater amounts of the ATP units of human energy. Voila! Exercise forces the muscles to generate more ATP, a physical basis for human energy. Exercise increases energy for necessary metabolic needs. Is it possible that the mitochondria continue to increase output of ATP once the exercise ceases?

Mars Hill and Long Covid

There is a story in the Christian Bible where the great missionary Paul finally made it to Athens, a great center of Greek thought and philosophy. He had a desire to share the Christian faith with the Greeks in hopes they would turn to Jesus.

> Tidbits:
>
> In Acts 17:28, the Greek word for "live" is *zao*; for "move" is *kineo*; for "have our being" is *esmen*. *Esmen* is also used later in the same verse as Paul is quoting certain Greek poets who have said that *"For we also are His offspring"*—"we are" is *esmen*. *Esmen* seems to indicate the totality of our existence, our consciousness, our life-force, our vitality; the wholeness of our soul and body and spirit and mind and thought and feelings and inner heart and outer heart.

Holy and Wholistic Health!

As Paul was addressing the philosophers and thinkers at the regular place of oratory and debate—the edifice known as the Areopagus located on Mars Hill—he made the following statements: *"God, who made the world and everything in it...He gives to all life, breath, and all things...He is not far from each one of us; for in Him we live and move and have our being..."* (Acts 17:24-28).

For in Him we live and move and have our being.

Segue to Long Covid (not a smooth segue; the next two paragraphs are mostly a repeat from an earlier section on breath). For all who have been infected with the Covid virus and have survived, many have fully recovered with no ongoing symptoms; others continue to experience residual symptoms (at some level) as a result of being infected with the virus. These residual symptoms have been termed Long Covid. I am not an expert in acute Covid or Long Covid; many others have studied Long Covid and have good data and understand it more thoroughly than me.

> **Pearl:**
>
> For in God we live (breathe) and move (energy, muscles, weakness) and have our being (our existence—soul and spirit and body and mind).

When I do read about the syndrome called Long Covid, it seems as though at least three areas are often involved: the strength (energy and muscles), the brain (brain fog, sleep, anxiety, mental/mood issues), and the breath (shortness of breath and other lung sequelae). Other symptoms and organ systems are often affected by Long Covid (such as heart issues and blood clots to name a few), but the three areas initially mentioned stick out to me as being significant symptoms often experienced.

Data and understanding of Long Covid is still, scientifically speaking, in the early stages. Time will undoubtedly reveal clearer understanding of Long Covid and hopefully helpful interventions.

Any natural-based and/or soul-based and/or spirit-based interventions

Muscles

> **Personal Tidbit:**
>
> My wife and I are just now getting over our first bout with the Covid virus, most likely the Omicron variant. The following is our experience (thus far). During the acute phase (days 1-3), we experienced mild typical flu-like symptoms, relying on lots of sleep, nutrition, more sleep, orange juice, more sleep, lots of prayer(s), and some zinc gummies from a good friend. Brain focus and concentration were difficult (similar to other types of feverish infections in the past). During the subacute phase (days 4-10), most flu-like symptoms resolved, but we had partial loss of smell and taste, occasional cough and nasal discharge spells. I was able to work remotely from home, and my brain focus and concentration was mostly normal. We still relied on lots of sleep and rest (no exercise), orange juice, nutrition, and lots of prayer (by us and others), and Bible meditation. Incidentally, a rapid nasal swab was still positive for me at day 5. During the post-acute phase (days 11 and beyond), symptoms were 99% resolved, except I can tell my energy reserve is not 100% of usual (on this day 16). We still have occasional paroxysms of cough/runny nose with smell/taste mostly resolved. Rapid Covid nasal test was negative at day 11 of symptoms. We have mostly returned to normal routines (daily prayer, Bible meditation, nutrition, plenty of sleep, normal work schedule with normal mental effort, lots of sunshine bathing, and fresh air). I have slowly started increasing my daily walking routine, and my energy seems to be increasing daily. Hopefully, these trends will continue over the next few days and weeks until all symptoms totally resolve (and maybe even better than pre-Covid). My wife and I have been blessed...

for Long Covid that can help (1) our lungs breathe, (2) our muscles release energy for strength, and (3) clear out brain fog and mental sluggishness and mood/thought dysfunction—are welcome to help improve and hopefully overcome the Long Covid symptoms.

What's With That Cough?

After being over Covid, I still at times have episodic paroxysms of cough/runny nose spells, but these episodes are not specific to Covid (for me).

For years, after I was over the acute phase of any upper respiratory infection that had affected my upper bronchial/respiratory passages, it was not uncommon for me to have occasional spells of coughing and runny nose—especially when I get hot, laugh, sing, or even recline backwards in a recliner or lay flat in bed with my face to the sky. It seems as though the now-resolved infection sensitizes the upper respiratory airways in a manner similar to when a nasal allergen swells up nasal mucosa and causes the nasal passages to get stuffy and/or run. These post-infection paroxysms of cough will eventually resolve (will eventually become non-sensitized). And, I'm sure if I took an inhaler or a brief course of steroids, these cough paroxysms would resolve sooner. Note: Steroids are an anti-inflammatory agent, seeking out and calming down bodily inflammation wherever bodily inflammation can be found.

No Bones About It

Closing out this section on BONES—diminished muscle mass can lead to diminished energy and can lead to experiencing poor health. Diminished or malfunctioning muscle tone can lead to poor muscular balance.

After a Theology Break interlude in the next section, the chapter following will discuss the importance of muscle balance, energy balance, homeostatic balance, and overall balance to our health.

Theology Break

Energy and life-force. Living in good health means **living in a state of energy and vitality** absent of disease and dysfunction, producing **maximum well-being** now and for many years to come (my definition). Anything that promotes and produces energy contributes to good health.

Energy is physical (ATP), and physical energy affects the invisible soul (nephesh), the well-being. And, humans are created as soul-spirits that can become spirit-souls (the goal of Jesus and Christianity). Soul is body-soul and soul-spirit...body-soul-spirit...spirit-soul-body. Anything that increases energy will affect every part of the human and their health. Three parts. Three points stick out to me.

First, the obvious to me: Anything that increases physical energy...ATP...such as exercise...increases the overall energy of the person. Second, it seems intuitive that anything that enhances the soul—mind, will, emotions, thoughts—might have the ability to increase overall energy, perhaps enhancing physical ATP production? Phrases such as "such-and-such brought me great joy and pleasure and re-invigorated and refreshed me" or "so-and-so is hilarious and recharges my batteries."

Verse:
The famous Psalm 23 states, *"...He restores my soul..."*

Another verse:
Recall that Proverbs 3:8 says relying on God and His wisdom will bring health to the body and strength to the bones.

> ### Energy Bible Verse:
> "*The Everlasting God, the Lord, the Creator of the ends of the earth, does not become weary or tired...He gives strength to the weary...to those who have no might He increases strength...those who wait on the Lord shall renew their strength...they shall run and not be weary, they shall walk and not become faint (or weary)*" (Isaiah 40:28-31 NKJV and NASB).
>
> ### Another Spirit-Energy Bible Verse:
> "*But if the Spirit of Him who raised Jesus from the dead dwells in you, He who raised Christ from the dead will also give life (zoopoieo) to your mortal bodies through His Spirit who dwells in you*" (Romans 8:11). *Zoopoeio* is the Greek NT word used in this verse and is translated in many ways, including to give life, invigorate by spiritual power, to restore, and to give increase of life, including increasing physical life.

Could such soul-type experiences actually enhance the production of ATP? I wish I knew how to measure ATP levels.

Now for the third, the spirit. As energy is a central, key component to good health, not acknowledging the role that the spirit can play would be irresponsible and shortsighted. A Christian-based spirit-soul has all of the resources of God and His Spirit to increase energy. A Christian who has the life of Jesus inside of them, in their spirit, is in union with God, as described in 1 Corinthians 6:17: *"But he who is joined to the Lord is one spirit with Him."*

> ### Rest Verse:
> "*Come to Me, all who are weary (and tired)...I will give you rest...you will find rest for your souls...*" (Matthew 11:28-29 NIV and NCV).

Learning how to draw on all realms of energy—from the natural, physical, soul, relational, and spiritual—will increase energy. If there was a quantifiable way to measure ATP in the body, I suspect that all of these energy sources would increase ATP. An increase in energy can help improve the symptoms of the syndromes that have low energy

Theology Break

> **Tidbit:**
> Recent research has focused on sleep and rest disturbances as potentially being a key in causing fibromyalgia.
>
> **Eye-Opener:**
> I once had a friend who was almost physically disabled from fibromyalgia. She began sleeping better, healthier, and almost all of her symptoms resolved. In her case, she told me that she started sleeping better after releasing forgiveness to a relative that had abused her.

or no energy, such as chronic fatigue or fibromyalgia. No matter what is causing fatigue or lack of energy, anything that infuses energy into the body can improve the symptom reality of low energy.

Faith-Energy Connection

In human biological systems, energy is a key to good health and proper functioning. Energy can be referred to as both a noun and a verb (energize), meaning it is a substance and is a substance that produces action. Solid and "do-able" at the same time.

> **Verse:**
> *"Now faith is the substance of things hoped for, the evidence of things not seen"* (Hebrews 11:1).

A related somewhat synonymous term in the spirit-soul world is faith.

The word *faith* is often used as a noun to denote a person's religious beliefs or the religious system that a person belongs to; for instance, someone might say, "I am of the Christian faith."

> **Another Verse:**
> *"Now faith comes by hearing, and hearing by the Word of God"* (Romans 10:17).

However, I believe there is a better explanation of the word *faith*. In the reality of the Bible-based spirit-soul, faith is a concept, a substance, a reality (noun)

Holy and Wholistic Health!

> ### Terms:
> The term *Rhema* is when one receives a specific, Holy Spirit-focused word from the general *Logos*, the totality of God's Word, the Bible. One might say that a Rhema word came alive in their spirit while meditating on the general Logos, the Bible.
>
> ### Personal Tidbit:
> So many times in my life, I have been at a crossroads of needing direction, needing to know the next step, needing to know which way to go in business or in family or in finances or any area of my personal life. And then...one word from God and...VOILA! A portion, a piece, a chunk, a unit even the size of a mustard seed of faith was suddenly there, providing real direction and, inherent in the substance of faith, was the energy and ability to act on it!

that can produce action (verb). Faith is a key reality to help determine a Christian human's success and guidance and provides for their life and the energy to carry out said guidance.

> ### The Small Things:
> *"He who is faithful in what is least is faithful also in much...and if you have not been faithful in what is another man's, who will give you what is your own?"* (Luke 16:10)

The substance and reality of faith can be imparted by different means; one of the key ways is by reading God's Word (Bible) and receiving it with an open heart; said another way—hearing a word from God.

Faith energy combined with actual muscle/physical energy is a win-win combination for good health and well-being.

Faithfulness Has Benefits

Another angle on the concept of faith is the reality of being full of faith that produces consistency in commitments—being faithful (faith-full). To be full of faith is to be a person who is faithful to show up and follow through in a marriage relationship or a friend relationship; will follow through on a job commitment; will follow through on their word or on

Theology Break

a promise that was made. Faithfulness in all of life is a desired character trait.

Long-term faithfulness in a job will often lead to advancement and promotion. A long-term trusted friend or neighbor might be privy to information that others are not. Long-term faithfulness that has produced trust in a marriage often leads to each person disclosing themselves to the other in the deepest and most intimate ways.

> ### Secret Pearls:
> *"The secret things belong to the Lord our God, but those things which are revealed belong to us and to our children forever..."* (Deuteronomy 29:29).

The Lord likes to reveal Himself at deeper levels and in more intimate ways to those who have been and/or are learning to be faithful back to Him.

The NT describes faithfulness as a fruit of the Spirit (Galatians 5:22), evidence of the new life of God's Spirit at work inside a person. Like all fruits, faithfulness over time in commitments is not present at the beginning of a growing season; faithfulness, like fruit, is developed over time by abiding and remaining in a healthy and vital relationship with God. Faithfulness develops and grows by staying intact with the vine—soft, tender, dependent, and pliable.

BALANCE

Balance

"The Balance of Life"

Balance is a buzzword in healthcare. Balance of homeostasis. Balance of muscles and posture. Balance of the whole of man—holistic, wholistic—in spirit, soul, mind, emotions, thoughts, social relationships. Balance of living life, balancing work with family with friends with pleasure. For good health, it is necessary to have, in general, overall balance and, in specific, balance in many areas.

Please Make the World Stop Spinning

"I lost my balance and fell down." The type of balance that is postural muscular balance, allowing a person to stand and walk without falling, is perhaps the most common usage of the word balance. Along with muscular weakness and frailty causing someone to fall, both of which will be discussed in later sections, it is not uncommon for someone to take a tumble because of dizziness, vertigo, or feeling light-headed.

Dizzy Woozy Light-headed Vertigo

Dizziness can be defined as a sensation of spinning around and losing one's balance. Vertigo is a closely related term. Vertigo is a type of diz-

> **More Dizzy Terms:**
> Associated terms and symptoms would include feeling light-headed, faint, weak, woozy. Nausea and feeling queasy are commonly associated symptoms. Isn't this a lovely discussion? Hope you're not eating right now.

ziness that creates the false sense that you or your surroundings are spinning or moving. None of these sensations are pleasant. I detest these sensations with a passion and try to avoid them at all costs.

> **Tidbit:**
>
> You might remember the semicircular canals from biology class as those three loop rings oriented in three different spatial planes. Whereas the cochlea coils on itself and resembles a snail, the semicircular canals look like, with a little imagination, a piece of modern art or a gyroscope.

The dizzy-vertigo-light-headed woozies are a common reason people lose their balance and fall—or just feel miserable or feel like they're going to pass out even if sitting or lying down.

These sensations of being off-balance can be caused by many things including heart problems or brain problems or from being dehydrated or anemic (just to name a few). However, a commonly blamed reason for vertigo would be a disturbance, an imbalance, in the inner ear.

The inner ear is made up of two main functions. One is for hearing and involves the cochlea as an endpoint of the auditory nerve. The auditory nerve is a branch of cranial nerve number 8 and is a key transmitter of outside sounds for hearing. The cochlea has a distinct appearance that kind of looks like the coil of a snail.

Cranial nerve number 8 has another functional branch known as the vestibular nerve. The vestibular nerve hooks into the semicircular canals, the other part of the inner ear, which if not functioning properly can cause dizzy vertigo.

The three loops of the semicircular canals with different spatial orientations are key to a human possessing the ability to sense

> **Perception Definition:**
>
> Proprioception is the perception or awareness of the position and movement of the body. Proprioception is the formal term for spatial awareness and balance. It is intricately linked with the semicircular canals, the vestibular nerve, and the occipital lobe of the brain.

Balance

where they are in space and if they are moving and, if so, what direction they are moving in. They are also key to maintaining spatial, postural balance at all times.

The semicircular canals are, of necessity, very sensitive. If they become disturbed in the slightest, such as if a small piece of cellular debris accidentally floats into one of their open, fluid-filled ends, a dizzy-light-headed-vertigo wooziness often ensues. These attacks are often in modern vernacular referred to as inner ear spells.

A disturbance of the inner ear causing imbalance and any form of dizziness is often termed vestibulitis or labyrinthitis. A common form of inner

Personal Tidbit #1:

I remember one morning seeing my wife get up out of bed and immediately fall back into bed with her "head spinning" furiously (not literally spinning like in the movies; she was just extremely dizzy to the point of not being able to stand). Before she stood up, she felt fine. Apparently, when she stood, she had an immediate inner ear disturbance—perhaps a piece of cellular debris floated into one of her balance canals? She stayed in bed lying very still for about an hour, and then got up and went on about her normal day with no more dizziness.

Personal Tidbit #2:

I discussed in a previous section developing spells of vertigo in the height of the Covid pandemic in late summer 2020. I was dumbfounded and ready to see a doctor for a full exam and testing. Then, one day I realized that the spells seemed to be connected to (1) inhaling Lysol-type disinfectants and (2) when I was in a tight, enclosed space. Voila! I was overdosing my system by sniffing too much Lysol that was exacerbated by claustrophobic situations. After backing off on unnecessary air disinfectants, the vertigo spells and claustrophobic tendencies went away! Healed! Miraculous! (Full disclosure—I prayed for healing also!)

Holy and Wholistic Health!

> **And Also:**
> Claustrophobia is an extreme or irrational fear of confined places. In my case, I would point out the word "fear" (-phobia) in this definition. Fears were running rampant in the height of the pandemic. Perhaps overall fear also played a part in my dizzy spells...
>
> **And Another Thing:**
> *"I sought the Lord, and He heard me, and delivered me from all my fears"* (Psalm 34:4). I'll take the removal of dizzy spells any way I can get it!

ear disturbance is BPPV—benign positional paroxysmal vertigo. BPPV is more common as people age and often shows up as a brief, temporary dizziness when the head is moved rapidly or in a certain direction.

Roller Coasters Don't Bother Me...

I remember my good friend and me riding the Orient Express roller coaster at Worlds of Fun in Kansas City approximately 10 times in a row before feeling a little "off." The Orient Express spun and twisted and looped upside down in two-barrel rolls at high speeds. Exhilarating! I was about 20 years old...and then I got older. Things changed. I changed. I now avoid all roller coasters at all costs. Things that spin and loop and go fast now disturb my inner ear balance almost immediately, produc-

> **Sorry Kids:**
> To give equal time to the Six Flags theme park in St. Louis...At about the age of 40, when my kids were still at home, I decided to man-up and ride a coaster with my son. We had a full breakfast, got to the park when it opened, ran to the Mr. Freeze coaster, and expectantly jumped in the front seat (why not, right?). We blasted off, and I was doing fine until...I realized this particular coaster stops in mid-ride and goes backward on the track. Uh oh! I completed the ride without hurling my greasy breakfast (a miracle). I wobbled off and, in genius fashion, rode another coaster trying to push my way through the voice of wisdom that was welling up within me telling me to stop.

> **(Cont):** After getting off the second coaster, I was extremely sick and dizzy, nauseated and woozy, off-balance and vertiginous. Somehow, I slowly made my way to a park bench to "sleep off" my inner ear drunkenness sensations. I insisted the family go on without me and enjoy their day—being the man that I am. I didn't know whether I would die (felt like it) or would be thrown out of the park for apparent (non-alcoholic) drunkenness. After about three hours, the sensations slowly began to dissipate, and I found my legs and caught up with the fam and—you guessed it—sat WITHOUT MOVING in the kiddy pool waterpark for the remainder of the day. Never again, roller coasters!
>
> ....
>
> ### Did I Mention I'm Thick-headed?
>
> A year or two later, I decided I would totally override the Lord's voice of wisdom and man up again and ride a coaster with one of my kids at Silver Dollar City, a local theme park. This particular coaster was similar to Mr. Freeze at Six Flags, except it did not reverse and go backwards. I can do this, right? After waiting in line for what seemed like forever...probably 1-2 hours...I parked my tushy in the coaster seat and...before they strapped me in with the crossbar...I heeded the voice of the Lord that was now screaming at me in my inner man and promptly jumped up and out the other side of the coaster car, apologizing to my daughter that she would be riding alone, wishing her a good ride, and telling her I would see her when her ride was over.

ing the aforementioned unpleasant sensations. I jokingly tell people that after about the age of 35 all my sphincters loosened up (insert surprised shocked emoji face here).

How Many Senses Do We Have?

It has been routinely acknowledged that humans have five basic senses: seeing, hearing, feeling, tasting, and smelling. Back to how important balance is. Because proprioception balance is so integral to the normal functioning of a human and involves perception and sensation, it has been suggested that proprioception be considered one of the basic human senses, being the "sixth sense" (haha), the "body awareness" sense. It has even been proposed that the closely related vestibular movement be added as the seventh sense of humans, being the "movement and balance" sense. Makes sense to me (sorry about that).

How Is Tinnitus Pronounced?

Some pronounce tinnitus with the accent on the second syllable, making it rhyme with laryngitis. Others say that the proper annunciation is to put the emphasis on the first syllable and accentuate the "Tin-", giving the word a much more proper and fancy sound. Whichever is correct, I pronounce tinnitus "ringing in my ears."

> **Definition:**
> Tinnitus is a sound that is heard within the head or ear(s) when no external sound is present. There are many descriptions of what the phantom sound may sound like...ringing, whistling, buzzing, chirping, hissing, humming, roaring, even shrieking.

All I know, after getting a middle and inner ear infection in my left ear at around the age of 47, I often have had a strange and unusual hum, a high pitch, in that ear which comes and goes, waxes and wanes...a classic presentation for tinnitus. The good news—it has lessened over time, and I have adjusted to it, which is common, only hearing it if I stop and focus. And sometimes not even hearing it then! The attenuation adjustment of not hearing it is good, since there are very few good scientific treatments that are proven effective. I'm sure it's not in any way related to all the loud music I have enjoyed listening to all my life, right?

> **Ringing Ear Tidbit:**
> I have tried some different supplements and treatments that are purported to help tinnitus, all to no avail. Perhaps I didn't try the right ones? What has seemed to help most, along with time and attenuation, is having it prayed for multiple times.

Aging, Reserve, Margin
"The Inevitabilities of Life"

It has been said that the normal aging process is a loss of physiologic reserve. Physiologic reserve can be defined as the ability to carry out normal biological activities under stress. Aging results in an accumulation of cellular damage in the body that is not being effectively cleared from the body; the body is not getting properly renewed or restored (thanks, AAFP, 2/15/21, p. 218, Vol 103 Number 4).

A similar concept relating to physiologic reserve is biological margin. A loss of physiologic reserve and biological margin make it difficult for the body to compensate for the moment-to-moment challenges that the body faces (such as when a routine DNA mutation causes a rogue cell...a monster...known as a cancer), and the body's normal surveillance system fails to detect and eliminate the problem. A loss of physiologic reserve interferes with normal homeostatic balance.

Frailty

Frailty is a recognized geriatric syndrome, a term often used to describe general decline as one ages. The decline often includes diminished mus-

> **Tidbit:**
> Sarcopenia is a medical term used to describe the general loss of muscle tissue as a natural part of aging (sarco- refers to muscle and -penia refers to loss of or a lesser amount). A goal of good health is to prevent sarcopenia and frailty and all other associated manifestations of physical weakness.

Holy and Wholistic Health!

> **Bible Tidbit:**
> In the Bible, the term "flesh" sometimes refers to human tissue (OT Hebrew *basar*) such as Genesis 2:21 where God *"caused a deep sleep to fall on Adam... and He took one of his ribs, and closed up the flesh in its place..."* Or the word flesh may have a spiritual meaning, emphasizing man's fallen nature without Jesus. The NT Greek word *sarx* is used both to describe physical, meaty flesh and is also sometimes used to describe man's fallen soul-spirit nature without God.

cular strength and energy, poor balance, decreased physical activity, exhaustion, cognitive decline, and weight loss. Geriatricians—medical experts in caring for the elderly—categorize an elderly person as being either frail or pre-frail or not-frail based upon their assessments.

Not all elderly people are destined for frailty. This book is written to attempt to prevent frailty—to stay not-frail—and to improve the health of those experiencing frailty.

> **Geriatric Health Hope:**
> A favorite verse of mine as I become older than I used to be and looking ahead, closing in on senior status, is Psalm 92:12-14: *"The righteous shall flourish like a palm tree, he shall grow like a cedar in Lebanon. Those who are planted in the house of the Lord shall flourish in the courts of our God. They shall still bear fruit in old age; they shall be fresh and flourishing..."*

It seems as though weight loss in the context of frailty is probably a cycle that feeds back on itself. In other words, weight loss will include a loss of muscle mass with a resultant lower level of energy, ATP and protein production and a diminished appetite. Low energy and low protein lead to not exercising and not lifting weights to increase muscle mass, resulting in further weight loss and low energy and an increase in frailty.

Staying Fresh

To re-quote one of my favorite verses, Psalm 92:14: *"They shall still bear fruit in old age; they shall be fresh and flourishing..."* Another version says, *"They are ever full of sap and green..."* and another says, *"They shall be fat...*" and another "*...virile still in old age.*" Lots of saying the same thing from many angles. I love it!

One of my favorite authors is Mark Batterson. Mark is a pastor in Washington, D.C., and a prolific writer. I make it a point to read one of his books every summer; this is good for me. It is one of my good health habits.

I have shared one of my favorite Bible verses, Psalm 92:14; now I will share one of my favorite Mark Batterson quotes: "At some point, most of us stop living out of imagination and start living out of memory. Instead of creating the future, we start repeating the past" (from his book *The Circle Maker*). Batterson notes that this tendency can be shown as actual anatomic brain changes that are confirmed with neuroimaging evidence on brain scans.

Upon writing this paragraph, I am 58. I have noticed that, as the years pass, it seems to become more natural for me to lean toward a negative perspective in situations and conversations. I have noticed it is easier for me—a Christian believer who has a born-again spirit renewed daily by God's Spirit and God's Word—to gravitate to being negative, grumpy, complain-y (not a real word), whiney (a real word), rigid, and stiff in viewpoints...maybe even cynical...and perhaps all in the auspices of wisdom. Perhaps the focus of my wisdom insight today will be the government...or taxes...or technology...or the internet...or the news...or healthcare...or my aches and pains...or the next generation...or that person who did me wrong...or how that person "should have done (insert something here) a different way." The list of topics is endless for my seasoned wisdom.

I know a few good examples of people who are more seasoned in

> ### Flourishing Tidbits:
> The OT Hebrew Bible has multiple words for flourishing including *para, parah,* and *raanan*. I love the definition of these words: to be luxuriant, green, budding, sprouting, blossoming, fresh, fruitful...and all in my older age...all by loving Jesus with all my heart, soul, mind, and strength and by being planted in the house of the Lord!

Holy and Wholistic Health!

age than me who have stayed fresh and flourishing in mind and spirit and soul and imagination. Their bodies might have aches, pains, scars, and malfunction, and yet, they are positive and a joy to be around. They are full of forward vision, not just living out of the past. This is my intentional goal as I get more rings around my trunk. It might not be easy to stay vibrant and fresh, but I am determined...

Longevity

"The Span of Life"

Often, when I pray for people, I will pray a blessing over them that they will live to be 120 with good health and a sound mind. According to the Bible, Moses lived to be 120 and *"his eyes were not weak nor his strength gone"* (Deuteronomy 34:7 NIV). God said that *"...his days (mankind's lifespan) would be one hundred and twenty years"* (Genesis 6:3).

When I pray this prayer of a 120-year-long life in good health and a sound mind (2 Timothy 1:7), the response is often that they're not sure they want to live that long, usually due to an expected chronic disease affecting the physical body (such as a stroke) or a chronic mind and brain problem (such as dementia or Alzheimer's). They don't want to go to nursing homes. I get all that; I don't want that either. But that was not my prayer for them.

The Blue Zones

Dan Buettner, a *National Geographic* Fellow and *New York Times* bestselling author, has co-authored a documentary and a book called *The Blue Zones*. In the Blue Zone study, five geographic areas on earth were identified where people tend to have long lifespans in good health, typically living to be over 100 and with their mental faculties intact. These five areas were the Nicoya peninsula of Costa Rica, the Japanese island of Okinawa, the Greek island of Icaria, the Italian island of Sardinia, and the Seventh Day Adventist city of Loma Linda, California.

Holy and Wholistic Health!

Dan and his colleagues studied the lifestyles of these people—in all five Blue Zones—to try to find the common denominators among all five groups that might be universally applicable for all people to be able to live a long and healthy life.

As I learned the Blue Zone principles for longevity, I realized two things. First, the Blue Zone principles tend to line up very well with the current evidence from the latest studies for good health and long life. Second, and most striking to me, the Blue Zone principles tend to line up with God's Word (the Bible) very well.

In no particular order, I will now describe the habits of Blue Zone longevity.

Make family a priority. Blue Zone inhabitants tend to have a strong priority on regularly spending time with family. The younger generations welcome the older generation into their homes; nursing home living tends to be almost non-existent. The Blue Zone elderly tend to be physically healthier and mentally sharper as they age with their social skills intact.

Of all the Blue Zone principles for long life, this one seemed to have one of the strongest correlations from the Word of God: *"Honor your father and mother...that your days may be long, and that it may be well with you..."* (Deuteronomy 5:16). This is one of the ten commandments, the only one with a promise—the promise of long life.

Another Blue Zone principle has a striking parallel with another of the ten commandments. Most Blue Zone participants **attend religious services regularly and make faith a strong foundation in their lives.** Deuteronomy 5:7 says, *"You shall have no other gods before me,"* and Deuteronomy 6:2 says, *"...that you may fear the Lord your God, to keep all His statutes and His commandments...you and your son and your grandson, all the days of your life, and that your days may be prolonged."*

Another of the ten commandments is *"Observe the Sabbath day, to keep it holy, as the Lord your God commanded you. Six days you shall work, but the seventh day is the Sabbath of the Lord your God. In it you shall do no*

Longevity

work...that your (servants) may rest as well as you" (Deuteronomy 5:12-14). Blue Zone inhabitants have found ways to **take time out of their lives to regularly de-stress and slow down life's pace.** For instance, the Seventh Day Adventists regularly take a sabbath day off from work, which serves as a powerful stress reliever, helping keep inflammation in check and adding joy to their lives.

Most of the Blue Zone inhabitants **eat mostly a plant-based diet with beans, whole grains, and vegetables making up the majority of their intake.** The Adventists are vegetarians. The other Blue Zones allow meat into their diets, but it is not a regular daily fixture, as it often is in the rest of the world. Genesis 1:29 says, *"And God said, 'See, I have given every herb that yields seed which is on the face of the earth, and every tree whose fruit yields seed; to you it shall be for food.'"* Interestingly, when God allowed meat and animal products into the human diet after the flood in Genesis 9:3 (*"Every moving thing that lives shall be food for you...I have given you all things, even as the green herbs"*), the extreme longevity of early Genesis began to decline.

Other Blue Zone health behaviors include **eating until 80 percent full and then stopping and moving naturally.** These amazing people that live longer lives have mastered the self-discipline of not over-eating. (The Bible has a lot to say about gluttony, such as in Proverbs 23:21 "*...the glutton will come to poverty.*") And the Blue Zone inhabitants were not gym rats or over-exercisers; they often were shepherds who walked many miles in a day and/or were gardeners and often just led an active lifestyle.

The Blue Zone centenarians had **a meaningful purpose in living** and, for the most part, were **socially engaged.** They had a reason to get out of bed—their purpose for being alive on the earth. They were not hermits, not known to complain. They were often fun to be around and sometimes were the life of the party. They tended not to be

> **Tidbit:**
> Another one of the Blue Zone longevity principles seemed to indicate that mild, moderate alcohol intake (wine) might be associated with a longer life.

grumpy and cantankerous—young people enjoyed being around them. They were known to have regular social meetings (apart from church and faith-based meetings) with friends and peer groups. The Bible does speak of *loving the Lord your God with all your heart, soul, mind, and strength* and *of loving your neighbor* (Mark 12:30-31)—this being the first and second in importance of all the commandments. God's Word also speaks of the importance of being hospitable and friendly (Romans 12:13; Proverbs 18:24) and of seeking first God's kingdom (Matthew 6:33).

Hormonal Balance

"The Rhythms of Life"

Humans have a nervous system—the brain, spinal cord, and peripheral nerves—that helps regulate all bodily functions via electro-chemical impulses. The human body has another regulatory system that also affects the entire body, the endocrine hormonal system. Endocrine hormones are molecules that are made in certain parts of the body (thyroid, adrenal, ovary, testicle, pancreas, pineal, pituitary), released into the bloodstream as chemical messengers, and accomplish work at different sites throughout the body. Hormones work with the nervous system to help monitor and regulate overall physiologic balance.

As such, if any of the hormones are out of balance—not working properly...too low or too high—all or a part of metabolism and homeostatic balance will be disrupted. Dysfunction. Disease. Trouble. Many patients come to my medical office because of hormonal problems or seeking out whether their problems are due to hormonal imbalances.

Rhythms, Patterns, Waves, Cycles

One of the great things about living in southwest Missouri is experiencing the four seasons. Almost on cue, winter turns to spring, spring turns to summer, summer to fall, fall to winter...a seasonal cycle, a rhythm. The timing may vary with minor differences from year to year, but the trend line of seasonal changes doesn't vary much at all.

The human hormonal system operates around a wonderful cycle called the circadian rhythm. Circadian means the tendency to recur naturally

Holy and Wholistic Health!

> **Weather Tidbit:**
> Southwest Missouri seems to be a battleground for the warm, humid southern Gulf air masses fighting with the drier southwest winds coming from the southern plains clashing with frigid northern weather fronts. Because of these air masses clashing, we can seemingly experience all the seasons in one day. The famous saying of the locals is, "If you don't like the weather, just wait a few minutes; it's gonna change."

on a 24-hour cycle. I remember when I first learned about the repeating periodicity of circadian rhythms, which especially pertain to endocrine hormone secretion into the bloodstream. The information about circadian rhythms explains some of the things I experience, such as why it seems so much easier for me to exercise around sunrise and why it seems harder to exercise around noon (obviously, that may not be everyone's experience).

> **Pitui-Tidbit:**
> The thyroid gland is a regulator of metabolism, maintaining homeostatic balance. It could be said, however, that the pituitary—that little pea-shaped gland at the base of the brain behind the eyes—is actually the master hormone regulator since it sends feedback signals to multiple hormonal glands, including the thyroid.

Endocrine hormones, such as the thyroid hormones, have an amazing and complex system of receptors throughout the body giving continuous feedback creating a continuous monitoring loop. The receptors continuously send "right now" information to the pituitary gland, which in turn signals the thyroid gland with the latest command to either lower or raise or maintain current thyroid hormone levels.

Taking time to learn about circadian rhythms can be helpful for daily health functioning as well as helping treat disease. Understanding circadian rhythms can give insight into such things as: the sleep-wake cycle; best times of the day to exercise, eat, or reproduce; body temperature; bowel movements; alertness; even why the blood pressure tends to rise in mid-morning and decrease later in the day. Understanding circadian timing is like catching a wave...more perfect timing...maximizing patterns of the body for maximum energy, health, and well-being.

Temperature Balance

"The Warmth of Life"

I am writing this section during the Covid-19 pandemic, and we are one year in. Body temperature—especially if elevated to the point of a fever—is always important; however, never more important than during this last year. "Do you have a fever?" has become a routine phrase before going to work or school, or to a restaurant, place of business, Walmart, grocery store, or to church...before going anywhere. Fever is one of the cardinal symptoms of Covid-19. Forehead thermometers, whether accu-

Definitions:

Technically, a fever is considered a body temperature 99.4 or above. The medical term for fever is pyrexia. Fever reducers such as Tylenol and ibuprofen are antipyretics.

More Fever Tidbits:

A fever can be generated internally or externally. Internally generated fevers would include infections and autoimmune processes and tumors and other disease-causing conditions. Other internally generated fevers can be caused by ingesting external things, such as certain medications, and due to medication reactions and vaccine side effects. Externally generated fevers would include being outside on a hot day or being in a heated tub or hot body of water for a period of time. Externally generated fever from exterior heat can eventually lead to internally moderated manifestations such as heat stroke and heat exhaustion.

rate or not, have become commonplace. I often jokingly tell someone as I am pointing a forehead thermometer at their head that it is a new form of brain scan. No one has yet been amused by my lame sense of humor. A body temperature in the considered normal range of around 97-99 degrees Fahrenheit optimizes human physiology and biochemical reactions. The temperature 98.6 is considered the gold standard of temperature normalcy. Many bacteria and viruses have a narrow range of viability, causing the human body under germ attack to swing the body temp low and then high (fever with associated chills), attempting to kill the would-be invaders. The debate rages on whether it is healthier to allow a fever to go unchecked or to lower a fever with medication, allowing the human victim to feel better and not dehydrate as fast. Pathologic infections are an ultimate imbalance.

Temperature and Infection Imbalances

I have noticed a few observations regarding body temperature that seem very consistent in my daily reality. To reiterate, the following observations have been repeatable in my personal experience; I'm not sure whether they are specific to me or apply broadly to others.

Observation #1: "I got a chill, and now I have pneumonia…or the flu…or (such-and-such) infection." I have heard the phrase, "I got a chill, and now I'm sick" so many times. You know what? It seems to apply to me. If my body temp drops for an extended period of time—such as getting wet in the rain in the winter, sleeping with a window open (or under a fan) in the spring/fall hot days and cool nights, or going outside in the winter without

> ### My ATLIT Observations:
> Infection-causing germs are potentially always nearby…at the door…being held in check by a healthy immune system. Anything that temporarily lowers the body's immunity—such as "getting a chill"—may allow the body's defenses to be stormed, allowing an illness-causing bug to get a firm hold and cause an infection. These observations are my ATLIT observations—"Anything That Lowers Immunity Temporarily." Not bonafide science; just what I personally seem to witness repeatedly.

Temperature Balance

> **ATLIT on Covid:**
> One week ago tomorrow (as I write this), I was feeling my normal healthy self and went out in the extreme cold for a 10-minute walk. The wind was very brisk, and I immediately started feeling a chill while walking, a different "coldness" than when I normally get chilly while walking. Within 30 minutes, I started to feel body aches and feverish. I was Covid positive.

shoes or socks, or not wearing socks to bed on a cold night—a few days later I often start to get a scratchy throat and runny nose, early signs that I may be coming down with a critter germ. I will call this observation my ATLIT (Anything That Lowers Immunity Temporarily) observation #1.

ATLIT Observation #2: I have noticed an almost reproducible, clockwork-like phenomenon in me—when the front of my neck is exposed to cold air or a cool breeze (such as when I am jogging on a cold day)—I have noticed that I almost always develop a scratchy, semi-sore throat. Hmm. I have no understandable physiological explanation why this happens to me. If I don't quickly remove the cold air on my neck, I tend to develop a full-blown throat infection. I will tie this observation into the next observation.

> **Family Tidbit:**
> My dad used to say that, if he didn't cover his ears when going out in the cold air, he would get sick. I have tested this hypothesis on myself, and it doesn't seem to hold up for me. In my pre-med days, as long as I had my neck covered with a scarf, I could ride my bike the two miles that it took to get to my classes...in temperatures below 32 degrees... with my ears uncovered and flapping in the breeze...and get no sickness. It seems as though uncovered ears in cold air would be one of my dad's ATLIT observations.

Time-out: Those Darn Colds. "Getting sick" is often the phrase used by many when becoming infected with the common cold, otherwise known in the business as an Upper Respiratory Infection (URI). The common cold (1) is common, (2) is irritating and annoying, (3) can become super-infected with other germs but most commonly just remains

Holy and Wholistic Health!

Common Cold Observation:

It has been interesting over the years to see how different individuals categorize and react to and treat a cold...interesting to hear the different names for the URI handed-down in families and people groups—"epizoodas" was one that piqued my curiosity from an old-timer from Louisiana—and to see the different remedies that either do help or reportedly help to cure the common cold and associated head and chest respiratory infections. We humans are funny creatures; we all tend to have an ongoing narrative story in our minds that helps to explain and make sense of our circumstances and the world around us.

Case In Point:

One dear elderly lady who was not a doctor-goer came in for an ear infection. As the story goes, she reported, "I haven't had an ear infection since I was a child...At that time, my granny had me urinate in a cup, and then she poured it into my infected ear...cured it, and I haven't had one since." I looked across the hall at the urine sample cups and wondered if she was planning on doing it again to get another 50 years free of ear infections. "It's a good thing you didn't have a sore throat," I responded snarkily. She didn't miss a beat and quipped back, "Oh, when we had throat infections, Granny would hang Grandpa's old sweat socks around our necks." I thought about another snarky comeback (might have actually said it): "Your granny must not have liked you very much," but I knew that Granny and her granddaughter (my current patient) were very sincere and affectionate about these memories and what they were saying. And, who knows—Granny might have been right! Let me know if you try either of these remedies and they work. Legal disclaimer: I am not recommending either of these treatments. Consult your qualified healthcare provider for healthcare advice.

as a cold, (4) is a virus, therefore not responsive to antibiotics such as penicillin or a Zpak, and (5) seems to go through a mostly repeatable pattern in me when I have an URI cold. For me, the first few days of a cold may be rough with a plethora of URI symptoms such as sore throat, runny nose, stuffy nose, body aches, fever, sneezing, watering eyes, and often lots of drainage down the back of the throat (post-nasal drainage). These initial symptoms might improve, but often I will have episodic recurrences of an irritating cough (especially at night) or runny nose/sneezing/watering eyes spells, and then feel fine with no symptoms. These paroxysmal episodes tend to hit later in the day when I'm tired and at night, or if I get overheated, or if I laugh. The residual inflammation in my lungs and nasal passages may linger for days or weeks before clearing up. Some medications can help resolve the ongoing non-infectious inflammation quicker after 2-3 weeks out from the start of the URI. (Note: The common cold URI symptoms listed above are exactly the same symptoms I have experienced with the Omicron Covid variant.)

On-Call Tidbit:

Back in the day during training when I was required to take my turn on overnight call for the hospital, I noticed that if I was up most of the night—often helping to deliver a baby or admitting new patients to the hospital—I would usually get (you guessed it) a scratchy throat and runny nose. Usually around 4:00 a.m. I also discovered the antidote. If I was able to go home after getting off call the next morning and sleep, I would wake up fine. If, however, my responsibilities took me back to the clinic and hospital for a full day's post-call work, it was not uncommon for me to be fully sick by the end of the workday.

Family Vacation Tidbit:

When the kids were younger and I was running a solo, self-employed family practice, vacations were considered a treasure and hard to come by. (Explanation: A potential definition of self-employed is no paid vacations and no paid time off.) To try and squeeze in just one more day of family vacation fun (often over a long weekend and/or a holiday weekend), we would usually leave after a long day of work, and I would attempt to drive all night, thus arriving at our destination as the sun was coming up the next day. Not smart on many fronts. I was usually able to pull it off when younger but don't even try now. Again, that wasn't smart or recommended. When we would arrive at our destination, my scratchy throat would dictate that I try to take a nap while the family did other things. Often, we were on a beach, which made my napping more feasible.

Holy and Wholistic Health!

ATLIT Observation #3: As I get older, I have noticed that a lack of healthy overnight sleep will make me feel "run down," which often leads to infections. Usually, as with keeping my neck uncovered in cold air, the first sign is a scratchy throat with a runny nose. However, if I am able to take an extended nap, I often nip the oncoming infection in the proverbial bud.

ATLIT Observation #4: Here's one that others might have different, even opposite, experiences with; yet, it seems to hold up in my world. Some of the sickest infections I have ever experienced came on me—better said, hit me like a truck—within 30-60 minutes after extreme exercising. I vividly remember once when I was on call in labor and delivery...up part of the night helping deliver babies...during a season when a vicious stomach virus was dropping the hospital staff like flies. I was proud of myself for avoiding this throne-hugging critter. (Bible note: Pride often goes before a fall.) After 7:00 in the morning and my call duties completed, I had the day off and planned on going home for the much-needed sleep. In my brilliance, I decided to stop by the fitness center to bust off a few calories before going home; Lord knows I needed to exercise. It had been quite a while since I had exercised. Well, you guessed it—after my intense treadmill session, I didn't even make it all the way home before making a visceral deposit beside the road; it was my turn. The stomach bug had its way with me.

> **Even More Proof Tidbit:**
> I recently was enjoying a beautiful autumn walk with my amazing wife. We were essentially done, and I reached for my phone and realized that I had lost it somewhere along the trail. Immediate panic ensued, realizing the ramifications of someone potentially picking it up and keeping it (data, security, etc.), not to mention just the hassle and cost of replacing it. I ran back at a faster pace than I normally jog, over the 2-3 miles, retracing my steps. No phone. I jumped in the car and calmed down and prayed and drove to the other trailhead where my wife was waiting. I noticed that during the drive I was experiencing a funny...odd...unusual indigestion. Long story short—(1) I found the phone (I believe the Lord tipped me off to its location...I walked right to it), and (2) I spent the night in the bathroom hugging the porcelain. I felt fine before my unplanned, frantic run to find my phone.

Temperature Balance

Overall, exercise is actually known to be immune-building. However, during the immediate post-exercise phase, there seems to be a temporary lowering of the immune system, making one vulnerable to any lurking germs. It has been my routine advice to patients who are fighting off an infection to stop all exercise for at least 5-7 days, take extra naps, go to bed earlier, sleep later if possible, and allow the body to focus all of its energy into fighting off the germ rather than diverting the body's precious energy stores to exercising. This advice has helped me get back to exercising quicker than if I just tried to soldier on through early infection symptoms, allowing a bacteria or virus an opportunity to drag on and become worse...allowing a scratchy throat to turn into strep throat...a cold into pneumonia...minor intestinal symptoms into—you guessed it. No explanation needed.

Others may have different experiences with exercising and fighting off germs. I honor that. Do whatever works for you. The proof is in the pudding. Jesus said be it done unto you according to your faith.

<u>ATLIT Observation #5:</u> And another thing...I have noticed that if I can keep my bodily core warm—my neck down to my lower abdomen...my vital organs—I seem to fight off infections better. If I know I am in an early battle with a critter (you know, the scratchy throat/runny nose thing), and then I pull out my multiple layers of shirts and coats...covering and warming my core...I usually reverse the infection curse. Maybe that's why old guys like me often have on an extra sweater or jacket when the teenagers are only wearing a T-shirt?

> ### Last Night's Example:
> Just last night, I found myself standing in wet clothes after an unplanned (by me) challenge to jump in a pool. I took the challenge. I stood around the rest of the night wet and feeling cold. I went home feeling a bit of a chill (it was August). I put on dry clothes and more layers than I normally would in August. I slept in those layers. I canceled my usual exercise for the morning. I woke up the next morning feeling fine!

> **Putting It All Together Tidbit:**
>
> As a result of all these ATLIT observations, when I am jog-running at any temperature from 65 degrees or lower, you might find me wearing three upper layers with the outer coat being extra fluffy and a scarf wrapped around my neck. And, all the while, the teenagers, millennials, and super-hip, serious exercisers are in their short sleeves and designer exercise apparel. It would be embarrassing to me if I actually cared what I looked like. Some have likened me to the Michelin Man advertisement (if you don't know what that means, think of a super-round Pillsbury dough boy...if you don't know what that means, you are probably one of the short sleeve teenage exercisers that always look at me funny). I like being able to exercise in extreme weather conditions...and enjoy it...and be warm and not get sick! I do think my exercise apparel has been a source of embarrassment for my family and friends.

Speaking of embarrassing my family with my exercise fashion, here's a good one. I discovered the perfect bliss of a certain brand of tennis shoe that perfectly works for me when jog-walking (its initials are New Balance cross-trainer 608XL). I can wear this shoe and have no untoward aches or pains. When I first started jog-walking...now 18 years ago...for frugality, I would put duct tape wedges on the heels of my shoes after the pavement wore the rubber heels down (after about 4 months of exercise with the new shoes). Duct tape would get me another 4-6 weeks in that pair of shoes. My family loved it (not).

More Micro Please

Having just discussed the common cold, I thought now would be a good time to discuss a few odds and ends about germs.

I took microbiology in college. A whole new microscopic germ-world was unveiled to my understanding. I can still remember the strange and odd smells from the petri dishes in the micro lab. Not pleasant. I also remember the in-depth realization of this new world of unseen bugs... proving by experiments all of the germs that can grow from the bottom

> **Neurotic Note:**
> Somewhere along my educational path, I learned the old-school psychiatric terms neuroses and psychoses; these generalized terms are no longer in favor and have been mostly replaced with more descriptive and modern and acceptable terms. Neurotic behavior tended toward irrational fears and extreme phobias with internalized worries and would include many of the anxiety and depression disorders. Psychotic behavior would include, as expected, all of the psychotic disorders that tend to have a break with reality as a component. (These explanations are very simplistic and could certainly be defined more accurately by a mental health specialist.)

of a shoe...or a coin...or a dishrag...or even freshly washed hands. If a microbiology student has paranoid tendencies, this new-found discovery of the unseen germ world might tip them into neurotic tendencies. And, one person's neurotic tendencies might be another person's good hygiene habits!

The microscopic microbiology germ-world includes many different strange and unusual entities such as bacteria and viruses and others. I will comment on only a few of these (usually) invisible invaders and let the infectious disease experts remain the experts.

> **Don't Try That:**
> To rid itself of parasites, the invertebrate, under-water dwelling nudibranch will perform autotomy—the act of self-decapitation; it will, within three weeks, grow an entirely new body free of parasites! (*Discover Magazine*, March/April 2022, p. 25)

That Went Viral

I find so many things fascinating as has been mentioned many times in this book. I find viruses fascinating. I am not an expert on viruses. But one thing I find fascinating is that different sources will classify viruses as a living entity (similar to the fact that bacteria are alive), and others do not classify them as alive. Fascinating! One reference called them "entities." Another actually called them organisms at the edge of life.

Holy and Wholistic Health!

> **Viral Tidbits:**
> Viruses include (to name a few) the common cold, the flu (influenza), most cases of nasal and bronchial infections, Covid, mono, hepatitis, HIV, chickenpox, shingles, rabies, measles, mumps, herpes...many stomach viruses... and many, many more. Some have suggested that at least 320,000 different types of viruses infect mammals. Note: humans are mammals.

Judge for yourselves as to whether viruses are living or nonliving. They can replicate (with the machinery of a host cell). They have their own genetic material...they can evolve...they do not have normal metabolic machinery...they do not generate energy...they are entirely dependent on hacking the cells of the host as a parasite.

> **Tidbit:**
> In modern usage, the term *antibiotic* usually refers to a medication that attacks and destroys bacteria; an example would be taking penicillin to cure strep throat by killing the strep bacteria. The term antibiotic essentially means anti-life (*bios* is a Greek term for life).

Because of the unusual structure and nature of viruses, it has been more difficult to design medications that can attack and destroy viruses. Of late, the viral researchers have been more successful in developing antiviral antibiotics.

When it comes to actual viruses, you do not want to go viral (sorry about that).

> **Covid Virus Spirit Tidbit:**
> The Covid-19 virus became a worldwide pandemic in the early months of 2020. It is believed to have originated in Wuhan, China (debatable and controversial and not the focus of this tidbit). There is a spiritual infection called sin that originated in the Garden of Eden for humanity and went viral. The whole human race has been infected with this pandemic infection. Sin is to the spirit what disease and injury and death is to the body. There is a cure for this spiritual infection—turning to the God of the Bible in repentance (repentance was discussed earlier in the Posture section).

Temperature Balance

What the Heck is That Thing?

So, last night I was surfing on my phone, and a pop-up news story popped-up (go figure) about Tardigrades. Tardigrade? Never heard of it. I diligently researched and found out—are you ready for this?

> Tardigrades, often called water bears or moss piglets, are near-microscopic aquatic animals with plump, segmented bodies and flattened heads. They have eight legs, each tipped with four to eight claws or digits, and somewhat resemble the hookah-smoking caterpillar from "Alice in Wonderland." Though tardigrades are disarmingly cute, they are also nearly indestructible and can even survive in outer space...There are currently about 1,300 known tardigrade species...Not all tardigrades live in extreme environments, but water bears are known for surviving extreme conditions that would kill most other forms of life, by transforming into a dehydrated ball known as a tun...have an unusual strategy for surviving harsh conditions: They enter an almost death-like state called cryptobiosis, expelling more than 95% of the water from their bodies, retracting their heads and legs and curling into a dehydrated tun...(Direct quotes from "Facts about tardigrades" by Alina Bradford and Mindy Weisberger published November 12, 2021 on the LiveScience website platform.)

Just for fun, you have got to look up pictures of these critters. Kind of cute and definitely scary-looking. And that's all I've got to say about that.

BEYOND

I have discussed wholistic health pearls pertaining to Breath, Blood, Brains, Bones, and Balance. There are other health pearls I would like to mention that do not necessarily fit into any of these categories. To maintain the letter B alliteration, I will lump these remaining health pearls in the category Beyond—beyond meaning encompassing everything else.

Tears

"When Life Leaks"

Note: Some of this was covered in an earlier section and will be rehearsed here.

Our eyes have a wonderful system to cleanse the outer layer of the eyeball from unwanted things (like dust, pollen, dirt) and keep the cornea layer moist at all times. Tears. Tears are produced in a gland at the outside top of the eye sac, a gland called the lacrimal gland. The tears pass across the eyeball and drain into a duct at the inner corner of the eye. This inner-corner duct (tube) is called the nasolacrimal duct and funnels the tears by gravity into the nasal passages to become part and parcel with nasal secretions (blubbering snot). A wonderful system of cleansing and moisturizing when it is working properly.

So, why is it that our eyes leak tears—cry—from the lacrimal gland when we are experiencing physical pain? Or emotional sadness or grief? Or extreme joy and happiness? I don't know why. One could postulate a parallel with the cleansing of the soul during emotionally tormenting tears, but that

> **Allergy Tidbit:**
>
> If the tear system is overstimulated with pollen or any allergy-provoking stimulus, the eye will over-tear and water excessively and itch. If the tear production is too much for the normal drainage into the nasolacrimal duct, the tears might overflow onto the cheek and run down the face. Allergy eye drops can help curb the excessive production of allergy tears.

wouldn't explain tearing during physical pain or extreme joy. Perhaps tearing-up in these situations is just a way for the body to have a physical release that might bring a soothing or comforting effect.

In fact, it is believed that a release of tears coincides with a release into the bloodstream of prolactin (a soothing and comforting hormone) and endorphins and enkephalins (the body's natural pain-relieving chemicals). Makes sense. It is also postulated that tears from peeling onions—"onion tears"—are a physical reflex response (similar to allergies) yet different from emotional tears; emotional tears produce more of a true physiological soothing and pain-reducing effect by releasing hormones into the blood.

Along this same line of thought, a distinction is made between what are called psychic tears (such as emotional pain tears) and reflexive tears (such as when peeling an onion). It is believed that psychic tears have higher levels of the feel-good chemicals than reflexive tears.

Good Grief

Just last night, I received news that a friend of mine had unexpectedly passed from this life, now face to face in the arms of Jesus. Immediately after receiving the news, after being shocked and deeply saddened, I began a grieving process. Tears. Prayers. More tears. Crying out to God. More tears. Songs. More tears. Grief is a real thing; and tears can be comforting, even healing. And, also, today is my wedding anniversary. Many swirling emotions today.

It is now widely accepted that there is such a thing as a healthy grieving process. A quick internet search can reveal the different theories of healthy grieving.

In contrast, there can be unhealthy grieving processes in which healthy stages of grief are not properly experienced; often, unhealthy grief is an unusually prolonged process in which the griever continues to feel very

Tears

real pain and sting and torment for many years after a tragic loss or tragic incident; a grieving, healing process that has malfunctioned. Stuck in a grief cycle.

Lamenting

Incidentally, healthy grieving is called a lament in the Bible. Proper and God-designed. Healthy grieving is good for health. It soothes the soul and helps the heart-soul-spirit heal after experiencing sudden loss or deep soul pain. The Book of Psalms in the Bible contains many heartfelt laments during times of agony; these particular Psalm laments are laments arranged in song form. Songs of lament.

The only way I have found true comfort during a grieving season is to turn to the God of the Bible. Here are a few of the grief-comfort verses I will soak in when in agony or grief or deep soul pain: *"God is our refuge and strength, a very present help in trouble"* (Psalm 46:1); *"...the Father of compassion and God of all comfort, who comforts us in all our troubles..."* (2 Corinthians 1:3-4 NIV); *"Blessed are those who mourn, for they shall be comforted"* (Matthew 5:4).

Having background worship songs playing that are focused on the divine lovers of my soul—God, Jesus, and the Holy Spirit—also helps me greatly while grieving. Any experiential manifestation of God's healing presence

> ### Doesn't Time Heal?
> There is a common phrase that says time heals all wounds. There is a lot of truth in that statement. In my own experience, in times of my deepest anguish of soul, the passage of time seemed to help apply a cathartic treatment to my raw soul. But, in one particular circumstance—actually in more than one circumstance—the torment wasn't going away; painful thoughts and memories continued to recycle through my heart and mind. I was spiraling down into a deep hole. And then, I realized—I was not applying the healing balm of the Lord's sweet truths to my damaged soul. When I started rehearsing and praying God's loving truths and promises into my situation(s), over time, my deep soul wounds healed.

helps soothe my troubled soul. Experiencing the personal presence of God—and the presence of others who care deeply, who might even cry with me...or just be there quietly—can have deep soul-healing effects.

Grandma's Grief

I remember a poignant story from my childhood. My uncle had unexpectedly passed away in a car accident in the prime of his life. To reiterate a truth that is very real to me, my uncle had unexpectedly found himself face to face in the arms of the lover of his soul, Jesus.

His mother, my grandmother, was immediately thrust into unplanned, deep shock and grief and sorrow (as we all were). My uncle was the baby of the family, the youngest of seven children. Grandma and my uncle were both Christian believers, and Grandma had a deep and enduring faith. At the time of my uncle's death, Grandma was a member in the same church as me and my family, so we had a mutual pastor. He was a godly man who was loved and well-respected. He was not religious, yet he knew the Lord at a deeper level than most Christians I had been around up to that time.

Many months later, I remember hearing Grandma recount this story (paraphrased): "As soon as Pastor heard the tragic news, he dropped all and came to the house...He came in and sat beside me and held my

> **OT Tidbits:**
>
> In the Old Testament, King David was called a man after God's own heart; however, in the early years of his life, David's life was constantly in danger from friends, family, and enemies. Many of the Psalms are David's emotional suffering laments set to music during really tough times in his life. In one of his extremely painful situations while being persecuted, David said that the Lord had put David's tears in a bottle (Psalm 56:8), inferring that God had seen and remembered every painful tear that David had shed. (See other references to David's tears and weeping in Psalm 30:6; 69:3; 126:5).

Tears

> ### When Life Leaks:
> *"To everything there is a season, a time for every purpose under heaven...a time to cry...the Lord is near to the brokenhearted...blessed are those who mourn, for they shall be comforted"* (Ecclesiastes 3:1; Ecclesiastes 3:4 NLT; Psalm 34:18; Matthew 5:4). When life leaks, the Lord is near; when tears flow, a portal to heaven has been opened.

hand...just sat there holding my hand...without saying a word...silence...for an extended period of time. His presence and silence meant more to me than anything else I remember from that awful time..."

Inflammation

"The Swelling of Life"

Inflammation is one of the hottest topics in current health research. (Note: That statement is a bit of a pun since inflammation is usually warm; most of my puns are accidental.)

I remember studying musculo-skeletal inflammation in med school. Inflammation, such as when an ankle is sprained and swells or when a cut on the finger gets red and puffy and tender, was explained as the body's normal initial process of healing an injury or skin laceration. A good thing. A healthy thing. A normal thing.

> **Personal Example:**
> I remember playing pick-up basketball at the outdoor courts in college. I was driving to the basket for (hopefully) a layup and...POW! BAM! Instant pain. I twisted my ankle and wrenched it into the ground while running at full speed with all my weight. Well, in those days I was young and tough and ignorant (ignorant meaning not knowing the correct thing to do). I did all the wrong things. As the normal inflammatory healing response started, I decided it would be good if I kept playing on it (you know...walk it off) and did not elevate it; I went home and put heat on it. All the wrong things. I put the normal inflammatory response into overdrive and, by morning, my ankle was the size of a large grapefruit. *And* extremely painful. I went to the ER and found out it was just badly sprained (not broken), and most of the extremeness of it was self-inflicted. I turned what would probably have healed in a few days (normal inflammation) into a three-month healing process (extreme inflammation).

The problem with musculo-skeletal inflammation of an injury is there are times when the normal immuno-healing inflammatory response goes into overdrive and is excessive. The ankle gets too big. The cut on the hand gets puffy, red, and infected.

Too Much of a Good Thing

When the immune system mobilizes to begin healing an injury, it sends many healing inflammatory substances (such as cytokines, white blood cells, bradykinins, eicosanoids, prostaglandins) to the injury site, and these substances begin their tissue-repair processes. Along with the musculo-skeletal inflammation that can be driven into overdrive and cause problems…a good thing turned into a bad thing…there are other ways the normal inflammatory immune system can be harmful.

Autoimmune: The immune system provides surveillance to the body, identifying and neutralizing or removing foreign or harmful things that have entered the body. For example, when the neck glands swell up as the lymph nodes neutralize a throat infection, sometimes the immune surveillance system misfires and begins to attack normal tissue, causing an autoimmune damaging process. Think rheumatoid arthritis, lupus, asthma, eczema, psoriasis, many thyroid dysfunctions, and many other conditions. The body literally attacks itself. Thank God for steroids, the naturally occurring hormones made in the adrenal gland. Steroids can be used—by the body naturally or medically when treating with compounds such as prednisone—to help calm down autoimmune over-inflammation. However, too much of any good thing, including steroids, can prove harmful and have its own problems.

Heart: All of the risk factors for heart attacks such as smoking, diabetes, high cholesterol, obesity, and high blood pressure, contribute to heart disease by causing physiological inflammation in the blood vessels that supply blood to the heart muscle. Suffice it to say that inflammation in the heart arteries can result in producing plaques that either block the artery directly or by breaking off a small piece, an embolus, that travels downstream and eventually plugs an artery that is too small for it to pass through. Heart attack!

Inflammation

<u>Nutrition and Gut:</u> Recent health research has focused intently on a concept of certain foods or types of foods being inflammatory to the inside of the gut, especially to the intestines. This inflammation at the surface of the intestines causes an irritation that affects proper absorption of nutrients across the intestinal lining, allowing the gut membrane to leak chemicals across and into the bloodstream that would otherwise have been kept filtered inside the gut (outside of the bloodstream). This condition has been described as leaky gut syndrome and is being studied as possibly being a root cause of many conditions.

<u>Brain:</u> It is hypothesized that inflammation crossing the blood-brain barrier and into the tissue of the brain may be a root cause of many degenerative brain processes including many forms of dementia.

Sensitivity

Well-known effects of musculo-skeletal inflammation include redness, swelling, warmth, and pain.

With inflammation, the injured area (such as a paper cut) becomes tender and sensitized. Many of the inflammatory mediators sensitize the nerve endings of the affected area. Pain! If the area accidentally comes into contact with certain substances such as salt water or rubbing alcohol—ouch! The area is now overly sensitized in ways that it wasn't before.

> **Medical History Tidbit:**
> Heat (calor), pain (dolor), redness (rubor), and swelling (tumor) are clinical symptoms of inflammation as defined in the first century AD by the Roman scholar Celsus.

> **Personal Tidbit:**
> I had a wonderful dad and was very grateful for how he and my mother raised me. One thing, however, I did not appreciate was my dad's theory that if an open cut was not bathed in rubbing isopropyl alcohol...well, it just had to be soaked in rubbing alcohol, or it wouldn't heal properly and might

> **(Cont):** get infected. It is true rubbing alcohol kills almost all germs. I'm just glad I have discovered there are other ways to clean a sensitized wound that do not provoke as much pain as rubbing alcohol. Note: Dad even used rubbing alcohol as an aftershave application. When it came to rubbing alcohol, he was 100% all in; when it came to rubbing alcohol, dad was one tough guy.

Soul Sensitivity

Humans can become physically sensitized to injuries and irritations through the biological inflammatory process. It is also possible for humans to become sensitized in their souls and their emotions. Psychological sensitivity can be a good thing, such as being very in-tune with the hurts and pains of others. Compassion, care, concern...such as when Jesus was moved with compassion to heal others (discussed previously)... are all aspects of healthy psychological soul sensitivity.

A different aspect of soul sensitivity is also a reality. Past emotional hurts and emotional trauma, which all humans go through, can sensitize a person...even allowing an individual to become psychologically over-sensitized...over-inflamed...to similar stimuli that caused the trauma. Sort of a parallel process of the immune response becoming overstimulated and

> **Inflammation of the Soul:**
> Much has been written on negative and unhealthy emotions affecting human physiology, factoring into certain disease processes. Two related emotions that can be quite harmful are bitterness and resentment. It is important to keep all sources of unhealthy smoldering inflammation out of the body, such as when a low-grade dental infection might contribute to heart disease. It is also imperative for humans to keep all smoldering unforgiveness, bitterness, and resentment at bay...gone...none. I, for one, do not want to take risks with my health by allowing soul-inflamed emotions to linger. I can't stress enough how important it is to keep all yuck and muck out of the soul heart and the biological heart.

Inflammation

causing harm; a person's overly-sensitized emotions can trigger physiological and psychological harms. PTSD. Panic attacks. A person smelling a certain odor they are previously sensitized to triggering a noxious, nauseating response. A psychologically over-sensitized person can experience biological trigger responses from their mind and emotions that might be mildly annoying...or incredibly dysfunctional...or even dangerous.

A lighter-side personal example of soul sensitivity: When I was a teenager, I went through a dark, tough time emotionally and spiritually. I was simultaneously heavily into the music of the day, the classic rock music of the 70s and 80s. I came through that incredibly painful time and received wholeness in my heart, mind, emotions, and spirit. Jesus helped me. However, to this day, whenever I hear some of those 70s and 80s songs—such as background music playing in a restaurant—it is not uncommon for me to have an immediate negative emotional response. I am sensitized to those songs in a negative way. My wife will often hear the same songs that cause me angst and say how much she likes those songs; in other words, she is not sensitized in a negative way to certain songs as I am.

> **How True:**
> *"See to it that...no poisonous 'root of bitterness' springs up and causes trouble...and by this many become defiled..."* (Hebrews 12:15 ESV).
>
> **Time-tested Pearl:**
> *"Keep your heart with all diligence... for out of it spring the issues of life"* (Proverbs 4:23).

Relationships
"The Connections of Life"

As was discussed in an earlier section entitled "Longevity," Dan Buettner, a *National Geographic* Fellow and *New York Times* bestselling author, has co-authored a documentary and a book called *The Blue Zones*. In the Blue Zone study, five geographic areas on earth were identified where people tend to have long lifespans in good health, typically living to be over 100 and with their mental faculties intact.

Buettner and his colleagues studied the lifestyles of these people—in all five Blue Zones—to find the common denominators among all five groups that might be universally applicable for all people to be able to live a long and healthy life. Of the nine habits of these "longevitarians" (obviously my word, just made it up), at least two of these are directly related to relational, social connections. These two relational Blue Zone habits for longevity include (1) making family a priority and (2) attending religious services regularly (making faith a strong foundation in their lives).

Covid Connections?

Relationships are based upon social connections, specifically, a good and healthy relational connection between two people. Relational connections can be individual (one-to-one) or in a group setting. Healthy relational social connections that might foster healthy long-life...in the Blue Zone...will undoubtedly include both individual and group social interactions (family and spiritual groups, see above). I think some would accuse me of having a firm grasp on the obvious in this regard.

Holy and Wholistic Health!

Enter Covid-19, which in my world, became significant March of 2020. Another firm grasp on the obvious—overall, Covid did not foster broad, healthy, social relationships. Quarantines...lockdowns...illness...masking...social distancing. To be fair, some people would argue that some of their inner-family relationships became stronger due to forced closeness of interactions day after day...and some that love the Zoom-style platforms might argue that their world of relationships expanded. I am happy for all in which the Covid era strengthened their social world.

> **Health Hugs:**
>
> According to *Discover Magazine*, a six-second hug can help prevent chronic illness and infections and act as a form of "stress buffering" and also release the feel-good hormones oxytocin, serotonin, and the endorphins (March/April 2022, p. 14).

However, I believe for most people, Covid moved the social and relational scale in the negative direction (just like it did the actual weight scale of those who gained their "Covid 20" pounds).

This book is about any and many things that can foster good health for the whole man—spirit, soul, body, social, relational...thriving in every way. I continually see new scientific studies (not just the Blue Zones) claiming the health benefits of strong and vibrant relationships. A person may be healthy in body and even some in spirit, but if the social part of their soul is not thriving, they have an imbalance. And imbalances will always eventually reveal themselves in one way or the other.

Levels of Relationship Connections

Now that I have established that some of my insights are "having a firm grasp on the obvious," I would like to state another: There are different levels of relationships, different levels of social connections, that we humans have with others. Some relationships are quite superficial and probably should be...a business interaction, a wrong number on the telephone, picking up an item and returning it to the stranger who dropped it while passing you on the street. Not deep. Not designed to be.

Relationships

At the extreme far other end of a relational connection spectrum would be the intimacy shared between a husband and wife. Enough said about that.

Friendship and Intimacy

I have done extensive study into both the biblical and the cultural definitions of both the concepts of friendship and intimacy. It is quite an endeavor when learning all the different definitions of these two relatively common levels of relational connection. I will not try to rehash all the different definitional angles of these two words.

For instance, regarding intimacy, many acknowledge it is not just how a man might define it—focusing on the physical, sexual aspect. Intimacy also involves deep relational connections at the social, mental, emotional, spiritual levels...the totality of what people are. I agree wholeheartedly!

> **Friendly Tidbit:**
> And don't even get me started on the different perspectives people have on what being a friend involves. What I will say about friendship is that all the definitions are, for the most part, healthy and positive; on that most people tend to agree.
>
> **Friendly Verse:**
> *"A man who has friends must himself be friendly...but there is a friend who sticks closer than a brother"* (Proverbs 18:24).

Walking Together

I would like to, for good health, dive a little deeper into a few different, healthy relationship connections I see modeled by three of the main characters in the Christian Bible—and in the Old Testament at that.

The patriarch Abraham was one of the first figures who developed a deeper relationship with God than those around him. God came looking for Abraham early in his life, when he still lived with his dad and his name was Abram. I will not try to rehearse the entire story of Abraham

Holy and Wholistic Health!

> **Walking Together:**
> I equate Abraham's friendship with God on the same level with someone who has a very good friend, a very close friend, perhaps even a "best friend." It's not that others who were alive at the same time and before Abraham did not have relational interactions with God. They did, and they had. The difference is that the Abraham-God connection deepened to a level of trust and sharing hidden secrets with one another. Sounds like the stuff of deep and healthy friend-intimacy between two individuals. Most of our friend relationships that go beyond the superficial—to some level of commitment, trust, enjoyment, accountability, and secrets-sharing—would be categorized as this level of friendship intimacy, and it is valuable to our overall health! Said another way, this level of friendly intimacy is a good goal for the vast majority of our social friendships. Blue Zone science helps to reinforce this.

and all he is famous for; however, as Abraham and God's relational interactions developed over time, the Bible makes the claim at least in three different places that Abraham was a friend of God (2 Chronicles 20:7, Isaiah 41:8, James 2:23). To reiterate, what is significant about this is that no one at the time or previously in the biblical narrative had been called the friend of God.

Face to Face

As the OT Bible story continues to unfold, another central figure appears on the scene—the Moses of Egypt who became a deliverer of the Israelites from their hundreds of years of slavery. Moses appears in the Bible story many hundreds of years after Abraham. As before, I will not attempt to cover all of the things he did and is known for; that would take quite some time, for he was quite an accomplished person. The relationship aspect I would like to pull out of his narrative is that, not only was he the most humble man that lived (Numbers 12:3), which in and of itself is a most worthy and admirable attribute; he also had a close conversational relationship with the Lord. *"...The Lord spoke to Moses face to face, as a man speaks to his friend"* (Exodus 33:11). In verse 14 of the same chapter, God said to Moses, *"My presence will go with you..."* as they discussed the upcoming dangerous journey through the desert. Later in the same chapter, Moses is craving an even deeper relationship with God. He already has face-to-face interactions while in God's presence...he wants more. And he gets it!

> ### Face to Face:
> In my mind, if Abraham's relational connection with God has many similarities to a very close, personal friend, then Moses's relational connection with God is more of a family relationship...brothers, sisters, parents, children...a deeper level of relational intimacy and access to their presence than even most really good friends would have. Moses's level of relational friendship intimacy with God took it to the next level...more intimate, more presence. More of a personal intimacy in relationship bonding that we all crave and need, and it makes us healthy. Blue Zone science helps to reinforce this.
>
> ### Family Health Tidbit:
> Not only do the Blue Zone discoveries reinforce the health benefits of prioritizing family; I can hardly pick up any respectable health-based study that does not make claims and reinforce the health benefits of family-level relational closeness.

In the Arms of Another

I had an "aha-firm-grasp-on-the-obvious" moment recently. If I am in any group of people...and if I am abiding by what most would consider social and moral determinants...there should only be one person with whom I am able to have the deepest level of human intimacy possible—my spouse (hope that doesn't make you blush).

Segue to the third OT Bible character I would like to discuss—David. Otherwise known as King David. David shows up in the Bible story approximately 300 years after Moses. I will not attempt to re-tell all that David is famous for; like Moses, it would take too long. Most of his story is good and positive; some is not good and not positive.

Holy and Wholistic Health!

I want to focus on the relational connection aspect between God and David. The Bible says he was a man after God's own heart (1 Samuel 13:14). I have meditated on this phrase at length and studied it from different angles. One thing that was certain of David—he continuously and passionately pursued an intimate relationship with the God of the Bible. In essence, like a smitten and mesmerized lover, he constantly went after God and His heart...all that God is.

David was a musician and a lover. His music helped fuel his passion. He wrote many songs to God including love songs. His son Solomon wrote the raciest love book in the Bible, the Song of Solomon. David was a whole-hearted lover of God.

In the Arms of Jesus:
Some say that the best married couples start off as friends. When two people are in a romantic, love relationship and experience that level of deep connection in an ongoing way—and if they are practicing their connection properly, especially within the moral constraints of God's ways—they will (1) be the closest of the close as pertains to relationship in spirit, mind, emotions, heart, and body (wink); (2) possibly bear fruit from their relationship closeness (including children); (3) hopefully enjoy this level of exclusive intimacy connection; and (4) probably live longer, if the latest scientific research is true.

Lover Pearl:
As mentioned under good friend intimacy and family level intimacy, I regularly read studies that purport the health benefits, especially longevity, of a healthy and thriving spousal relationship! Interestingly, it seems as though many of these studies claim that this level of relational intimacy seems to benefit the man more than the woman. Huh. I could expound on this with lengthy speculations but will probably just leave it at that.

Relationships

Except to Say...

I couldn't resist being in a discussion about romantic intimacy relationships and not saying another thing or two (insert heart emoji here).

As was briefly mentioned a few paragraphs ago, it seems as though I regularly read studies that purport the health benefits, especially longevity, of a healthy and thriving marriage relationship. This is not to focus on potential negative health benefits of not being in a married relationship but to try to help maximize the good health reality of those who are married.

> **Disclaimer Reiterated:**
> Any individual who is not married can experience all the same health and longevity benefits of an unmarried person. No guilt, no shame; not inferior or less than; no inferred poor health declarations to the single.

You Big Flirt

A Google search defined flirting as "to behave as though attracted to or trying to attract someone." In marriage, flirting can (and probably should) be a regular part of romantically interacting with each other. In a God-sanctioned holy devoted marriage relationship, behaving in a manner of being attracted and trying to attract the spouse is fun and continues to cement the emotional and physical and mental bonds between the two partners. Being the relationship guru that I am (smiley face emoji or confused face emoji here), I highly recommend ongoing flirting in marriage to prime the flourishing of the holy bond.

> **Flirty Dating:**
> Flirting in a courtship dating relationship might be fun and helpful as long as the two potential future-mate flirters know where their boundaries are. Enough said.

Then there is unhealthy flirting. Can I have another moment where I have a firm grasp of the obvious? Please indulge me. Unhealthy flirting might show up in many different circumstances. Some examples of inap-

One Thing Leads to Another:

As the very purpose of flirting is to attract or show attraction for another... that will, by design, probably lead to acknowledging of said mutual attraction...which will, by design, probably lead to some form of behavioral actions (gasp)...which, by design, is to envelop the heart's emotions. Said simply, flirting can lead to something good...marriage, intimacy in marriage—or something bad...sin. The Proverbs 4:23 verse *"Keep your heart with all diligence...for out of it spring the issues of life"* is a good one to memorize and rehearse regularly. For good health!

Can I Just Say:

In my opinion, it seems as though some humans who are considered more attractive, prettier, smarter, kinder, more sensitive, well-liked by all seem to have a harder time with inappropriate flirting and a harder time "putting their nickel down" by committing to one person in an ongoing monogamous relationship. The world around them tells them not to limit their options and lock-in to any one committed relationship. (See an earlier discussion under the heading "The Beauty and Pleasure of Holiness" in the "Theology Time-Out" section for further comments on holy and holiness.)

propriate flirting include making goo-goo eyes, using indiscriminate words, and/or making inappropriate gestures toward someone other than your own spouse...someone who is the mate of another person...or with a "player" (a person behaving as though attracted to an individual... but for amusement rather than with serious intentions).

Speaking of Potential

Segue. In the embryonic formation of a human, the human embryo goes through multiple phases and transformations before eventually emerging through the birth canal as a human discovering earth outside the womb. Along the embryonic pathway, the multiplying fertilized cells develop early on as stem cells. Embryonic stem cells are pluripotent, meaning that they have the ability—the potential—to develop into all the different specialized cells that make up the whole of a biological human. Amazing!

Relationships

> **Regenerative Tidbit:**
> A currently hot topic in healthcare is regenerative health, defined as the process of replacing or regenerating human cells, tissues, or organs (in order) to restore or establish normal function (thanks, Google). Without getting into potential ethical or moral controversies surrounding regenerative health, it is one practical application of stem cell realities.

Now You're Reaching

I see a parallel process in stem cell science and the human social maturation process. *"Are you kidding me?"* might be your thought right now...or perhaps you're thinking, *"This is going to be a real stretch."* You might be right. But here goes anyway. When a young person, say in their late teens or early adulthood, is told they have the potential to do anything...to be anything...to marry anyone...these statements may be (mostly) factual. Thoughts such as *don't limit yourself by committing to* (fill in the blank with a job, a relationship, etc.) often circulate in their minds. The rush of such potential might be exciting, even exhilarating!

Here's where the conundrum often comes in—as long as the person remains in a state of stem cell existence (they have great potential), their value is only potential, like the pluripotent stem cells in the embryo. When embryonic stem cells begin to differentiate into specific tissue cells, they are now actually usable. Now valuable to the body. The tissues now incorporate them into the purpose and destiny for which they exist.

For all stem cell to social parallel applications, I'll leave it up to the reader to connect the dots.

Detoxes

"Life's Cleansers"

Not in any particular order, here is a list of my favorite detoxes:

- Sleep
- Water (drinking water)
- Fresh air (including sunshine, nature)
- Elimination (bathroom necessities, smile face emoji)
- Exercise
- Prayer
- Sabbath observance
- Regularly worshiping with my faith community
- Intermittent fasting
- Bathing

That is my list. These are my favorites and are very effective to detox harmful or unpleasant things out of me.

A few points. Detoxing is closely associated with other concepts such as cleansing and replenishing. Also, some of my detoxes are daily rituals, while others are more weekly or bi-weekly.

Sleep, fresh water, fresh air, exercise, bathing, and healthy elimination are simple, inexpensive, and easily available for most. Healthy sleep is now known to cleanse the brain of cellular debris, hopefully helping prevent brain trash build-up that might lead to dementia. Fresh air and water cleanse the blood and lungs. Hopefully, fresh air is accompanied by sunshine and nature, both which have replenishing power. Bathing cleanses the skin. Exercise with sweat helps excrete toxins from our pores and generate energy. And elimination...bathroom duties (pardon the pun)... well, hopefully the detox power of those are obvious.

I intermittently fast regularly. It is believed that intermittent fasting leads to autophagy, the cells' way of breaking down poorly functioning cells

Urine Tidbits:

Urine is a waste-filled liquid of filtered toxins and metabolic waste excreted by the kidneys and eliminated through the urinary tract. A main excreted waste product is urea, an unneeded nitrogenous metabolic product of protein metabolism; urea is a main factor in the unpleasant smell of urine. Some say that it has an ammonia smell, ammonia also being a nitrogenous compound.

Dr. Clark Pee-arls? (sorry):

I regularly drink lots of fresh, filtered water. Guess what? The more water I drink, the more I have to "go." The more I drink water, the clearer and less malodorous is the urine, which makes me feel good that I am doing my part to cleanse and detox my body through the urinary system. Also, the more water I drink, the better I feel overall—more energy, less brain fog, able to process information and function at higher levels.

Poo-phoria (sorry again):

The obvious detox function of having a bowel movement should be obvious. Another well-being benefit of a good BM—most people feel better after having "dumped" out the unwanted and unneeded digestive leftovers. I have heard the term "poo-phoria" as a play on the word euphoria to describe the pleasant healthy feeling of being "lighter" after a BM. My dogs certainly seem to prove this concept as they like to run circles in the yard immediately after said deposits. (Note: I am so, so, sorry for all the junior high puns in this section...well, maybe not that sorry.)

and passing them from the body. (Note: I have written extensively on intermittent fasting in a short booklet titled *Waiting To Eat*.)

My Favorite Soul Detoxes

The soul is a scriptural concept that refers to the invisible-ness of a human—mind, emotions, and will. The soul's hard-to-touch qualities of being human are intricately interconnected with the touchable body. The invisible parts of the soul and the visible parts are only separable for the sake of discussion, like a living human's brain and heart are only temporarily separable for surgery (or dissection once the life has departed).

The concept of detox obviously insinuates removing toxins...poisons... substances that are harmful. Closely connected detox concepts are (1) cleansing (cleaning) and (2) replacing toxins with good, healthy things.

This brings me to my favorite soul detoxes:

- Prayer—helps detox harmful things that have built up in my soul and spirit and cleanse me with God's goodness, replacing toxicity with God's strength and joy.
- Weekly Sabbath Rest—detoxes and cleanses me from the busy-ness and over-commitments of life and helps my body, soul, and spirit recharge and renew.
- Regular meetings of worshiping with my faith community—detoxes and cleanses me from an overly toxic self-focus, replanting me outward in relationships and community.

Prayer is daily for me, scheduled in my morning quiet time and continued throughout the day. Sabbath rests are weekly, and faith community meetings are (at least) weekly. In contrast, the physical-focused detoxes described in the earlier blogs are daily.

Simple, easy, affordable, and all natural! A lifestyle of detox.

The Tortoises and the Hares

"Physiological Speeds"

Human physiology—the intricate systems and processes that make the human body function...live...be full of energy—I find it all very interesting.

I have come to a conclusion about physiology. Some bodily processes tend to respond and change very rapidly—the "hares" of physiology in reference to one of Aesop's Fables about a race between a rabbit and a turtle. The moral of the story aside (that the slow and steady tortoise won the race), some physiological processes change and respond quickly (hares), and other bodily processes move slowly (tortoises). For the sake of my amusement, I will mention a few of those here.

Fast-Moving Hares

From a physiological perspective and timeline, the following processes seem to change and respond quite rapidly:

- Blood pressure and heart rate
- Blood sugar and triglycerides
- Weight scales—on fad and restricted diets; often mostly shifts in water
- Most bowel infections

Slow-Moving Tortoises

However, other bodily processes tend to adjust and change more slowly. A few of the physiological tortoises would include:

- Weight scales—actual, healthy weight loss
- Waistline—perhaps one of the more accurate measures of true weight loss and weight gain
- Cholesterol levels
- Kidney function—creatinine and eGFR measurements
- Bone density
- Most bowel patterns (Note: Many BM rhythms can be shifted and adjusted over time with intentional diet and lifestyle disciplines.)

Esteem

"The Confidence of Life"

The definition of esteem is "to set a high value on; respect, admire, hold in high regard." Often, the term *esteem* is used when speaking of another person; for instance, "I hold them in high esteem." A similar phrase would be, "I hold them in high regard; I have great admiration and respect for them."

The invisible part of the soul of a person—the heart, mind, thoughts, emotions, and feelings—needs a confidence, a rock, a foundation in order to function properly. Without an inner confidence that is believed to be based upon something solid, the soul doesn't seem to do well.

> **Self-Esteem Tidbits:**
>
> A definition of self-esteem would include confidence in one's own worth or abilities; self-respect. A result of self-esteem means you mostly feel good about yourself.

Some mental health issues might be traced back, at least in part, to a lack of confidence. Many will put their esteem in their own abilities and understanding, thus the common phrase self-esteem.

I remember a time in my childhood and teen years that I lacked esteem. I did not have any confidence in myself or my abilities; I had no self-esteem. I did not have any confidence in most of the other people that I knew. I did not have any confidence or admiration or respect for most of what I saw in the earth and the created world. As a result—you guessed it—my mood and attitude were usually negative and hopeless. I was no fun to be around (a "Debbie Downer" to quote a common cultural phrase); and

Holy and Wholistic Health!

> **Bible Tidbits:**
> Many verses, especially in the Psalms and Proverbs, speak of *"strength failing... bones wasting away...groaning all day long...energy (vitality) drained away as with the burning heat of summer..."* (Psalms 32:3-5; Psalm 31:10; many other similar verses).

my stomach often hurt, and I often had a general feeling of uneasiness. I lacked confidence; I lacked any esteem in my life; my soul-body was not coping well as a result.

I was having a hard time finding a solid rock foundational substance that would give me confidence from the natural world or the soul world. And then, one day...I gave the Jesus-related Spirit world another try. Here's an amazing Bible verse (previously unknown to me) that I found: *"Grace and peace be multiplied to you in the knowledge of God and of Jesus our Lord, as His divine power has given to us all things that pertain to life and godliness, through the knowledge of Him who called us by glory and virtue, by which have been given to us exceedingly great and precious promises, that through these you may be partakers of the divine nature..."* (2 Peter 1:2-4).

When I discovered the previous passage in 2 Peter, what immediately stood out to me was the end phrase ***"you may be partakers of the divine nature."*** I was already convinced that without God, my own previous nature was not going to get the job done; it had only caused me much heartache and grief and poor health. This discussion of how man's spirit died and the soul was trying to run the show was discussed thoroughly in the earlier "Journey into Theology" section of this book.

> **Tidbit:**
> When I discovered the 2 Peter 1:2-4 passage, I had already had relational encounters with the God of the Bible and with Jesus. Something had happened inside of me. Something had changed. Many terms might be used to describe what had happened in me, terms and phrases such as I became *a new creation* or *born again*, or *I gave my life to Jesus* (and many other descriptive terms and phrases). All good, all biblically accurate. All I knew was that something was different, and it was good; all for the better!

Esteem

I was amazed. By becoming spiritually alive to God (becoming a spirit-soul to complement what I already was, a soul-body)…I could literally become a partaker of God's divine nature. If I could be in a state of spiritual union with God—partaking of His divine nature—I had finally found a stable and substantive substance to give me confidence to live life. I did not have to rely on simply feeling good about myself, which had

> **Tidbits:**
>
> The Gospel of John chapters 14-17 are an amazing source to find out about the concept of being in union with God and Jesus…being spiritually one…in essence, partaking of the divine nature (verses such as John 17:21).

proved to be wishy-washy and unstable. My soul could now thrive with a divine spiritual anchor. My body could benefit from this confidence, this divine nature. My psycho-somatic tendencies went away!

> **Term:**
>
> Esteem in God that gives me a healthy self-esteem and self-worth has been termed finding my identity in God. This is a good way to say it. By being a new creation person that is spiritually alive to God, I have an identity of value and self-worth; a healthy self-esteem.
>
> **Another Divine Reference:**
>
> When the great first-century Christian leader Paul was dialoguing with the philosophers in Athens, he made this statement: *"And He has made from one blood every nation of men to dwell on all the face of the earth, and has determined their pre-appointed times and the boundaries of their dwellings, so that they should seek the Lord, in the hope that they might grope for Him and find Him, though He is not far from each one of us; for in Him we live and move and have our being, as also some of your own poets have said, 'For we are also His offspring.' Therefore,* **since we are the offspring of God,** *we ought not to think that the* **Divine Nature** *is like gold or silver or stone, something shaped by art and man's devising"* (Acts 17:26-29).

Stress

"The Pressures of Life"

Another proof that I have a firm grasp on the obvious—life is full of stress. We all have stress in our lives. Life stressors...life's pressures...can be healthy and produce positive and beneficial results. However, when discussing stress from a health standpoint, the negative side of stress is usually described; negative stress can lead to many health symptoms and even to disease and dysfunction processes.

Blowing a Fuse

A human—body, soul, and spirit—is a miraculous, elegant, complex system. Hopefully, this book has shed some light on just how intricately designed a human being is.

> ### Healthy Circuits:
> If the spirit-soul-body circuitry of a person's life gets overloaded with built-up pressure, tension, and stress—and this is not dealt with regularly in a healthy way—the individual might metaphorically blow a fuse and start to develop resultant symptoms. Common manifestations of an overloaded or blown circuit might be a new or unexplained "tension" headache or upset tummy or bowel changes or elevated blood pressure, just to name a few. In the mental health world, the dissociative disorders might, at times, have circuitry overload as a part of the reason why they are manifesting during a time of high stress or severe emotional psychic pain. Other mental health syndromes might also have similar causation at times.

Holy and Wholistic Health!

As has been discussed many times throughout this book, if there is any dysfunction or imbalance or problem at any level of a human's person, symptoms and dysfunctions and diseases will often eventually manifest. This is the understanding behind the term psychosomatic symptoms and psychosomatic illnesses.

The Nervous Breakdown

Apparently, the healthcare system of yesteryear was quite different from the one of today. I remember hearing an elderly acquaintance telling me that, in days past, if they felt like they were about to have a "nervous breakdown"—a term that I have a hard time finding in modern psychiatric diagnostic manuals—they would call and inform their well-trusted doctor that they were going to check themselves into the hospital because they needed a few days off...from the world and all of its pressures and expectations...to avoid a nervous breakdown. In hindsight, not a bad idea. I guess I better not go there...

> **Straight from the Mayo Clinic Website:**
>
> "The term 'nervous breakdown' is sometimes used by people to describe a stressful situation in which they're temporarily unable to function normally in day-to-day life. It's commonly understood to occur when life's demands become physically and emotionally overwhelming."

Universal Tension

Life stressors could also be described as life's pressures. Pressure and stress, in physics terms, are intricately related to tension.

The universe is established on tension. Without tension in a bowstring, an arrow will not fly. Without the tension of different muscle groups, it is impossible to walk. Without chemical tension across a cell membrane, the heart muscle cannot beat. Without electrical tension between electrons and protons, there is no electricity, no lights, no kitchen appliances. Without rest, exercise destroys. Without exercise, rest destroys. Without play, work destroys. Without work, play destroys.

> ### Biblical Tension:
> Tension is present within the kingdom of God and the truths of Jesus. For instance, Galatians 6:2 says, *"Bear one another's burdens,"* and Galatians 6:5 (just a few verses later) says, *"...each one shall bear his own load."* Well, which is it? The answer is yes—both of these truths are true. There seems to be a tension between them. They are not contradictory...they are just both true. It is possible for me to only believe one of these truths and base my life on that one facet of truth. In the long run, I will not do well; I will have a partial foundation, not a full foundation.
>
> ### Foundational Tidbit:
> Partial foundations will crack and crumble over time. John 1:17 says, *"grace and truth came through Jesus Christ."* Jesus is fully grace and fully truth. Each of these truths are amazing in and of themselves. However, one without the other will give me a faulty foundation. Mark Batterson, author of *Whisper: How to Hear the Voice of God,* says it this way: "Grace says that I will always love you; truth says that I will always be honest with you (tell you the truth)."

Knowing that stress/pressure/tension is a normal part of being alive—and necessary for healthy living—I do not always run and retreat when stress surfaces, whether the stress is relational or financial or survival-related or health-related or work-related or God-related.

When two seemingly opposite forces are left side-by-side and tension is generated, power and movement are possible. Think of magnets. When power and movement are generated through tension, anything is possible.

> ### Healthy Spirit Tension:
> After many years of attempting to make the Christian Bible a linear, non-irritating, easily-explained narrative so as to not tempt my intellectual mind to reject the life-giving principles found within, I now endeavor to leave the truth tensions of Scripture side-by-side. I don't try to do away with one to establish the other. As a result, I have found a healthier and more robust spirit life that invigorates my soul-body.

Final Thoughts

Well, I hope this book has been informative...educational...enjoyable...or at least mildly entertaining in trying to delineate what is the essence of good health and how to live a long, happy, and healthy life with maximum energy and well-being. I hope the thoughts set forth in this book will help a person to live in a state of energy and vitality absent of disease and dysfunction producing maximum well-being now and for many years to come!

Perhaps a good way to wrap up this book is by sharing a phrase I love. An old preacher pastor had lived to a ripe old age and eventually passed away in his late 90s. Before passing on, when asked what the secret to his success in his long life and ministry was, he is quoted as saying, "Keep it simple, travel light, and don't sweat the small stuff." Well said! Having followed his life and ministry, I know he found the ability to keep it simple, travel light, and not sweat the small stuff—all by having a healthy relationship with Jesus.

*Reminder: The thoughts and opinions set forth in this book are not to be considered as medical advice or diagnosis or treatment. Be sure and consult your qualified healthcare provider for all medical and healthcare advice and diagnosis and treatment.

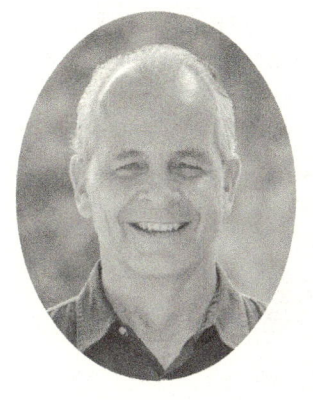

GUEST SPEAKER

Dr. Jonathan Clark, M.D.

www.jonathanclarkmd.com

Family Physician, Olive Grove Medical
Ordained Minister, Abundant Life Church

As a family practice M.D. for over 30 years and an ordained pastor since 2009, Dr. Clark passionately studies biblical truths and medical science so he can have a solid knowledge base to care for his patients and when speaking to groups. His teaching style reflects his fun-loving, humorous personality, while he imparts wisdom about living a healthy, whole life. He has witnessed advances in medicine and miraculous healings—both of which are created by a loving God. When speaking to an individual or a large group, Dr. Clark/Pastor Jon takes deep and sometimes complex truths and delivers them in a warm, comprehensible, compassionate way. His words from the Holy Spirit bring healing to the spirit, soul, and body. He is also in the early stages of forming an all-Jesus, without-walls Holistic Healthcare Collective consisting of medical providers from different healthcare streams who are committed to providing holistic healthcare centered around Jesus.

Topics:
- Dr. Clark's Experience with Intermittent Fasting
- Jesus-centered Wholistic Health
- Praying for Miracles
- Sleep and Memory
- Emotions and Heart Health
- Neuroplasticity and Brain Health
- Energy and Vitality
- Longevity and Aging
- Holistic Detoxing

Great for:
- Keynote
- Church Services
- Conferences
- Mission Trips
- Consults

For information about scheduling a consult visit with Dr. Clark, visit *www.olivegrovemedical.com.*

To inquire about Dr. Clark speaking at your event or to receive a free copy of Dr. Clark's e-book on intermittent fasting, *Waiting To Eat,* visit his website: *www.jonathanclarkmd.com.*

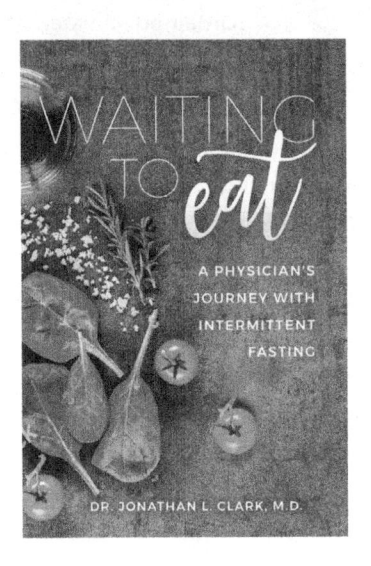

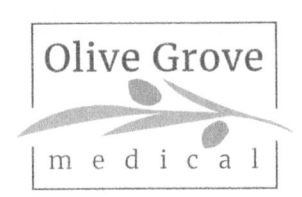

Made in the USA
Coppell, TX
02 January 2023